Patient C

A Dental Su

Patient Care
A Dental Surgeon's Guide

Crispian Scully
MD, PhD, MDS, FDS, MRCPath

Professor and Head of Department
Centre for the Study of Oral Disease
University Department of Oral Medicine, Surgery and Pathology
Bristol Dental School and Hospital
Lower Maudlin Street
Bristol BS1 2LY

1989

B·D·J

First Edition 1985
Second Edition 1989

ISBN 0 904588 23 8

Typeset, printed and bound in Great Britain by
Latimer Trend and Company Ltd, Plymouth

Preface to the First Edition

From the rather sheltered academic environment of the university, the graduate dental surgeon is thrown into the world to deal with often difficult and sometimes worrying clinical problems. Faced with making his or her own decisions, often with minimal background experience, and building relationships with patients and professional colleagues, the transition from being a student with few responsibilities, to a qualified dental surgeon can be traumatic. Enthusiasm is often at a maximum at a time when experience is necessarily limited: hopefully, the new graduate will have insight. Although a major change at this time of transition is from discussing the academic aspects of management to putting concepts into practice, documentation of the more practical aspects of patient management is not readily available. The dental surgeon who is a resident, working in a general hospital, or who is treating medically or physically handicapped patients is often made more acutely aware of these shortcomings. There may even be more senior members of the profession who, like me, find it difficult reliably to recall data from memory, particularly with the introduction of new drugs, new units, and so on.

The object of this book is to help in these situations by presenting some of the more practical aspects of diagnosis and management, mainly in note and tabular form, primarily for dental surgeons in hospital posts. It is a relatively brief synopsis, designed as a pocket companion or *aide-mémoire* that should complement the basic undergraduate training in dental surgery. The book covers many of the areas of dentistry that overlap with, or border on, other specialties in the field of medicine and surgery, but does not attempt to duplicate all the data already available in standard texts such as the medico-legal aspects of dentistry or details of operative techniques. The book should prove valuable to those working for Fellowships or other exams and also to senior students and auxiliary staff.

Crispian Scully
May, 1985

Preface to the Second Edition

In the five years since the first edition was written, dentistry has advanced rapidly, and the new five-year curriculum and almost inevitable mandatory vocational training should further improve standards in the UK. The first edition of this book appears to have proved useful and popular, but there is now a need to widen the remit and extend its usefulness to both hospital, general practice, and community trainees, as well as addressing the wider dental scene in North America, the Antipodes, Europe and elsewhere. I have therefore taken the opportunity to update and correct omissions and errors, and have included aspects of restorative dentistry relevant to this wider remit, as well as improving details on conscious sedation.

The cover shows dental care of an immunocompromised patient; these face masks are not routinely used on other patients.

Crispian Scully
1989

Acknowledgements

The foundations of this book were laid during my time as a resident, and inevitably the text reflects the views of the various surgeons, physicians and dental surgeons with whom I have worked. I am particularly grateful to Stephen Flint, Jane Luker, Stephen Porter and David Wiesenfeld, and my colleagues and friends in Bristol and elsewhere, who have advised and constructively criticised the contents.

I am also grateful to Margaret Seward and Sue Silver of the British Dental Journal, for encouraging me to write this second edition and particularly for agreeing to include the more comprehensive index which I had desired for the first edition. I am grateful to those who helped with the first edition and to John Wright and Sons and Professor R. A. Cawson for permission to use material from the first edition of *Medical problems in dentistry* in that text.

Contributors

The following members of staff of Bristol Dental Hospital and School have made contributions to the sections noted:

M. J. Griffiths, MB, BS, BDS, FDS, Consultant Dental Surgeon:
Radiotherapy Patients and Cytotoxic Chemotherapy

J. W. Ross, LDS, FDS, Consultant Oral and Maxillofacial Surgeon:
Maxillofacial Trauma

J. P. Shepherd, MSc, BDS, FDS, PhD, Senior Lecturer/Consultant in Oral and Maxillofacial Surgery:
Maxillofacial Trauma, Cryosurgery and Laser Surgery

C. D. Stephens, BDS, MDS, FDS, MOrth, Professor, Department of Child Dental Health:
Orthodontics

A. C. Watkinson, BChD, FDS, DRD, Lecturer in Prosthetic Dentistry and Dental Care of the Elderly:
Denture Care

Contents

1

History, Examination, Investigations and their Interpretations, and Dental Records

1.1 Oral history, examination and investigations

Dental history, examination and investigations are discussed in standard texts and summarised in Tables 1.1 to 1.6. It is useful to use diagrams to illustrate the site, shape and appearance of lesions (fig. 1.1). Tooth charting is usually carried out using the Palmer system, but is now changing to the FDI system (Table 1.1).

Table 1.1   The more commonly used tooth notations

Palmer	Upper
Permanent dentition	Right $\dfrac{87654321 \mid 12345678}{87654321 \mid 12345678}$ Left
	Lower
Deciduous dentition (anonymous classification)	$\dfrac{\text{EDCBA} \mid \text{ABCDE}}{\text{EDCBA} \mid \text{ABCDE}}$
Haderup	
Permanent dentition	$\dfrac{(8+)(7+)(6+)(5+)(4+)(3+)(2+)(1+) \mid (+1)(+2)(+3)(+4)(+5)(+6)(+7)(+8)}{(8-)(7-)(6-)(5-)(4-)(3-)(2-)(1-) \mid (-1)(-2)(-3)(-4)(-5)(-6)(-7)(-8)}$
Deciduous dentition	$\dfrac{(50+)(40+)(30+)(20+)(10+) \mid (+01)(+02)(+03)(+04)(+05)}{(50-)(40-)(30-)(20-)(10-) \mid (-01)(-02)(-03)(-04)(-05)}$
Universal	
Permanent dentition	$\dfrac{1 \;\; 2 \;\; 3 \;\; 4 \;\; 5 \;\; 6 \;\; 7 \;\; 8 \mid 9\;10\;11\;12\;13\;14\;15\;16}{32\;31\;30\;29\;28\;27\;26\;25 \mid 24\;23\;22\;21\;20\;19\;18\;17}$
Deciduous dentition	$\dfrac{\text{A B C D E} \mid \text{F G H I J}}{\text{T S R Q P} \mid \text{O N M L K}}$
Fédération Dentaire Internationale (two-digit)	
Permanent dentition	$\dfrac{18\;17\;16\;15\;14\;13\;12\;11 \mid 21\;22\;23\;24\;25\;26\;27\;28}{48\;47\;46\;45\;44\;43\;42\;41 \mid 31\;32\;33\;34\;35\;36\;37\;38}$
Deciduous dentition	$\dfrac{55\;54\;53\;52\;51 \mid 61\;62\;63\;64\;65}{85\;84\;83\;82\;81 \mid 71\;72\;73\;74\;75}$

Table 1.2   Investigative procedures in diseases of teeth

Procedure	Advantages	Disadvantages	Remarks
Percussion (tapping and pressure)	Simple. May reveal periostitic teeth	Crude	Teeth may be periostitic due to abscess formation. Maxillary teeth may be periostitic if there is sinusitis
Application of hot or cold stimuli to teeth	Simple	Crude. Heat or cold may be transferred to adjacent teeth	Cold stimuli may be useful to locate pulpitic teeth or exposed dentine
Electric pulp test	Simple	Unpleasant. May give false positives or negatives. Requires special apparatus	May be useful to locate pulpitic teeth
Transillumination	Simple. May reveal caries	Crude	Rarely used
Radiography	Simple. Can reveal caries and much pathology in jaws	Pulp exposures may be missed as view is only two-dimensional. Caries does not show well on extra-oral films	Simple periapical films are valuable. Bitewing films do not show the periapical bone (see Table 1.18)

1.2 General history, examination and investigations

These are discussed in standard texts, but the best way to acquire these skills is by sitting in on an examination carried out by a physician or surgeon. The medical history *must* be recorded (see Chapter 3) and sometimes a check list is useful (Fig. 1.2). Remember that it is the clinician's responsibility to elicit an accurate history; if that necessitates finding an interpreter, for example, then the clinician must arrange this.

The dental surgeon is expected to be able at least to record the 'vital signs' of temperature, pulse, blood pressure and respiration, and must be prepared to interpret the more common and significant changes. In view of the involvement in the management of patients with head injuries, you must also be prepared to assess the conscious state and neurological function, particularly of the cranial nerves. You should also be able to assess the patient's mood and general well-being, but if in any doubt, ask for advice. If you think the patient looks ill, he probably is.

Some particularly serious symptoms or physicals signs to be on the lookout for in dental patients are given in Table 1.7.

Table 1.3 Investigative procedures in diseases of the jaws and sinuses

Procedure	Advantages	Disadvantages	Remarks
Radiography (see Table 1.18)	Reveals much data not obvious on clinical examination	Specialised techniques may be difficult	Most useful views are panoramic, oblique lateral, occipitomentals
Computerised axial tomography (CAT scan) and magnetic resonance imaging (MRI)	Reveal data often not seen on clinical or conventional radiographic examination	Expensive and not universally available	Demonstrate both hard and soft tissues and give spatial relationships
Transillumination	Simple	Crude	May show fluid in maxillary antra
Fibre-optic endoscopy	Simple; good visualisation	Expensive	Rarely used
Bone biopsy	Definitive	Invasive	
Aspiration of cystic lesion	Simple	May introduce infection	May show presence of haemangioma. Protein content of cyst fluid may be of diagnostic value (protein levels below $4\,g\%$ in keratocysts)
Bone scan	Surveys all skeleton	Those of any isotope procedure	May reveal (for example) metastases

Table 1.4 Investigative procedures in temporomandibular joint disease

Procedure	Advantages	Disadvantages
Radiography	Simple. Can reveal much pathology	—
	Arthrography (double contrast) provides excellent information	Danger of introducing infection. Painful
	CAT scan provides excellent information	Expensive
Magnetic resonance imaging (MRI)	Provides excellent information without exposure to ionising radiation	Expensive and not universally available

Table 1.5 Investigative procedures in salivary gland disease

Procedure	Advantages	Disadvantages
Sialometry[a] (salivary flow rates)	Simple rapid clinical procedure which may confirm or refute xerostomia	Somewhat imprecise. Wide range of normal values
Sialochemistry	Laboratory investigation. Useful mainly in Sjögren's syndrome ($\beta 2$ microglobulin raised)	Salivary composition varies with many factors. Far less useful than blood and other tests
Blood tests	Simple and can reveal systemic disease (eg rheumatoid arthritis)	Will not usually reflect local disease of salivary glands
Plain radiography	Lower occlusal and oblique lateral or OPT may show submandibular calculi. Soft PA film may show parotid calculi	Calculi may not be radio-opaque. Sialography may be needed
Sialography	Useful to eliminate gross structural damage, calculi or stenoses	Time consuming and somewhat crude and insensitive. May cause pain or occasionally sialadenitis.[b]
Salivary gland biopsy	Labial gland biopsy is simple and may reflect changes in other salivary (and exocrine) glands. Major gland biopsy may be diagnostic in localised gland disease. Needle biopsy may be useful	Invasive. May give false negative in disease of patchy distribution. Major gland biopsy may result in facial palsy or salivary fistula
Scintigraphy and radiosialometry	Measures uptake of radionuclide[c] Radiosialometry more quantitative. High uptake (hotspots) may reveal tumours. Also demonstrates duct function and potency and gland vascularity	Expensive and with hazards associated with use of radionuclides. Taken up by thyroid gland; rare instances of thyroid damage
Magnetic resonance imaging, CAT scanning and ultrasound	Useful for investigating space occupying lesions	Expensive, and not universally available

[a] Stimulate parotid salivary flow with 1 ml 10% citric acid on to tongue; flow rates of less than 1 ml/minute may signify reduced salivary function. Alternatively, pilocarpine 2·5 mg IV may be used but is contra-indicated in cardiac patients or those with hypotension. Most centres use citric acid stimulation
[b] Combined sialography with CAT scanning may be useful in diagnosis and localisation of salivary gland lesions, particularly parotid neoplasms.
[c] Usually technetium pertechnetate

Table 1.6 Investigative procedures in oral mucosal disease

Procedure	Advantages	Disadvantages	Remarks
Biopsy	Gives definitive diagnosis in many instances	Invasive	Mucosal biopsies should be submitted for histopathological and often direct immunofluorescence examinations if a dermatosis is suspected (see Table 2.1)
Exfoliative cytology	Simple, non-invasive procedure	Of virtually no value in diagnosis of oral mucosal disease. Many false negatives	Biopsy has superseded cytology
Bacteriological smear and culture	Simple clinical procedure	Isolation of organisms does not necessarily imply causal relation with disease under investigation	Anaerobic techniques may be indicated in oral lesions in the immunocompromised host
Fungal smear	Simple clinical procedure	As above	*Candida* hyphae suggest *Candida* species are pathogenic
Viral culture	Simple clinical procedure. Often gives diagnosis more rapidly than does serology[a]	May require special facilities and may only give retrospective diagnosis. False negatives possible	Indicated in some acute ulcerative or bullous lesions. Serology should also be undertaken
Haematological screen; Hb, red cell and white cell indices	Simple clinical procedure	Detection rate may not be high	Essential to exclude systemic causes of oral disease, especially ulcers, glossitis or angular stomatitis (see Chapter 2)
Serology	Demonstration of a rise in titre of specific antibodies between acute and convalescent serum may be diagnostically useful. Specific tests available, eg HIV antibodies	Serum autoantibodies may not mean disease. Serum autoantibodies may be absent in pemphigoid. Diagnosis of viral infections is retrospective	Essential in suspected dermatoses, connective tissue disease, autoimmune or other immunological disorders

[a] Electron microscopy gives the quickest results.

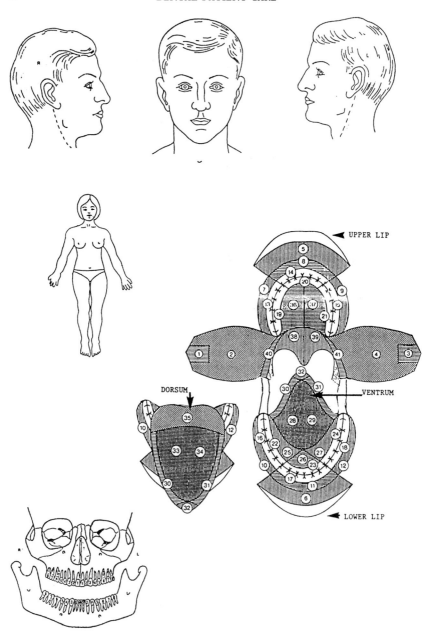

Fig. 1.1 Diagrams for outlining the site, size and shape of lesions.

		No: if YES, details of relevant medical history
CVS	**Heart disease,** hypertension, angina, syncope	
	Cardiac surgery, rheumatic fever, chorea	
	Bleeding disorder, **anticoagulants,** anaemia	
RS	Asthma, bronchitis, TB, other chest disease, smoker	
GI	Renal, urinary tract or sexually transmitted disease	
	Pregnancy, menstrual problems	
CNS	**Hepatitis,** jaundice, other liver disease	
	CVA, Multiple sclerosis, other neurological disease	
	Psychiatric problems, drug or alcohol abuse	
	Sight or hearing problems	
LMS	Bone, muscle or joint disease	
Other	**Diabetes,** thyroid, other endocrine disease	
	Allergies: eg penicillin, aspirin, plaster	
	Recent or current **drugs**/medical treatment	
	Steroids	
	Skin disease, use of creams or ointments	
	Previous **operations**, GA or serious illnesses	
	Other conditions (incl. congenital abnormalities)	
	Family RHM	
	Born, residence or travel abroad	
	Relevant questionnaire	

Fig. 1.2 Relevant medical history.

Table 1.7   Symptoms and signs of serious significance

Symptom or sign	Possible interpretation
Fever alone or with increased pulse rate	Infection
Fever with rapid, thready pulse, rapid breathing and lethargy	Serious infection; a 'toxic' patient
Fever with rapid, thready pulse and falling blood pressure	Serious infection and possibly septicaemia
Fever with thirst, lethargy, rising pulse rate and falling blood pressure, and falling urine output	Dehydration
Rising pulse rate and falling blood pressure	Bleeding, possibly hidden, eg into abdominal cavity; shock or anaphylaxis
Falling pulse rate and rising blood pressure	Rising intracranial pressure, eg intracranial bleeding
Absent pulse	Cardiac arrest
Irritability, vomiting and/or decreasing consciousness with or without other signs	Rising intracranial pressure or other causes of coma, eg hypoglycaemia
Fits appearing after a head injury	Brain damage or rising intracranial pressure
Severe headache, particularly if associated with neck stiffness, vomiting and drowsiness	Meningeal irritation, eg from meningitis
Cranial neuropathy appearing in a patient with head injury	Direct damage to nerve, or rising intracranial pressure
Stridor	Laryngeal obstruction, eg foreign body or laryngospasm
Wheezing alone	Bronchial or bronchiolar obstruction, eg foreign body or bronchospasm
Wheezing with collapse, falling blood pressure and weak, thready pulse with or without oedema	Anaphylaxis
Hyperventilation	Hysteria; pain; cardiovascular disease; neurological disease or metabolic disease
Dyspnoea	Respiratory disease or obstruction, or cardiac disease
Irregular respiration	Respiratory obstruction; brain damage; drugs or metabolic disorders
Persistent polyuria	Overhydration; diabetes mellitus; diabetes insipidus or hyperparathyroidism
Oliguria	Dehydration or renal failure
Collapse	See Emergencies (Chapter 4)

Standard forms will help with the symptomatic enquiries and with recording of data elicited by examination. See Appendix 1 for the various abbreviations used in clerking.

Taking the patient's temperature (Tables 1.8 and 1.9 show causes of fever)
(1) Leave the thermometer in place for at least 3 minutes.
(2) The normal body temperatures are: oral, 36·6°C; rectal, 37·4°C; axillary, 36·5°C.
(3) Body temperature is usually slightly higher in evenings.

Taking the patient's pulse (Table 1.9)

Sites
The pulse can be recorded from any artery, but in particular from (a) the radial artery, on the thumb side of the flexor surface of the wrist, (b) the carotid artery, just anterior to the mid third of the sternomastoid muscle, and (c) the superficial temporal artery, just in front of the ear.

Rate
Infants have a rate of 140 beats/minute, reducing to 60–80 beats/minute in adults. Pulse rate is increased in exercise, anxiety, fever, some cardiac disorders, hyperthyroidism and other disorders.

Rhythm
Should be regular; if not, ask a physician for advice.

Table 1.8 Causes of fever[a]

Inflammation	Infections[b]; connective tissue disorders; chronic granulomatous disorders (sarcoid; Crohn's disease); transfusion reactions
Neoplasms	Hodgkin's disease, etc.
Drugs	Methyldopa, etc.
Endocrine-metabolic	Thyroiditis; malignant hyperpyrexia
Thermoregulatory disorders	Midbrain, pontine or hypothalamic disorders
Other	Factitious fever; post-ovulatory (luteal) phase of menstrual cycle

[a]Transient pyrexia follows severe exertion, hot baths, etc.
[b]Chronic or minor infections in any patient, or other infections in the elderly or immunocompromised may not cause pyrexia.

Table 1.9   Changes in vital signs in patients with infection

| | | Changes associated with infection indicative of | |
Vital sign	Normal range	Mild to moderate infection	Serious infection[a]
Temperature*	35·5–37·5°C	37·5–39·5°C[b]	Above 40°C
Pulse	60–80/min	90–100/min[c]	Above about 100/min
Blood pressure	Systolic: 120–140 mmHg; diastolic: 60–90 mmHg	No change	If falling may indicate shock
Respiration			
Airway	Clear	Clear	If not clear
Rate	12–18/min	18–20/min	Above about 22/min
Rhythm	Regular	No change	Any change in rhythm or depth

[a] Admit to hospital. CNS changes are also indications for admission. These include decreasing consciousness, intensive headache with stiff neck and/or vomiting, eyelid oedema, visual disturbances
[b] If the temperature is above 38·5°C and a bacterial infection is suspected, consider taking blood cultures (Section 1.6)
[c] Often higher in children
*Oral temperature

Character and volume

These features vary in certain disease states and require a physician's advice (Tables 1.10 to 1.11).

Taking the patient's blood pressure

(1) Seat the patient.
(2) Place sphygmomanometer cuff on the right upper arm, with about 3 cm of skin visible at the antecubital fossa.
(3) Palpate the radial pulse.
(4) Inflate the cuff to about 200–250 mmHg or until the radial pulse is no longer palpable.
(5) Deflate cuff slowly while listening with stethoscope over the brachial artery on skin of inside of arm below cuff.
(6) Record the systolic pressure as the pressure when the first tapping sounds appear.
(7) Deflate cuff further until the tapping sounds become muffled (diastolic pressure).
(8) Repeat. Record blood pressure as systolic/diastolic pressures (normal values about 120/80 mmHg, but these increase with age (Table 1.12.)

Table 1.10   Common symptoms and signs of cardiac disease

Symptoms	Cardiac causes	Other causes
Breathlessness (dyspnoea)	Cardiac failure	Respiratory disease; anaemia; renal failure
Ankle swelling	Cardiac failure	Venous obstruction; renal failure; liver disease
Angina	Myocardial ischaemia in coronary artery disease	Other cardiac disease; severe anaemia
Palpitations	Often insignificant but may indicate cardiac disease	Tachycardias
Cyanosis	Cardiac disease including right to left shunts	Respiratory disease
Ankle oedema	Cardiac failure	Venous obstruction; renal failure; liver disease
Finger clubbing	Cyanotic heart disease	See Table 1.13
Abnormal pulse rate, bradycardia	Heart block	The elderly, athletes, drugs
Tachycardia	Cardiac disease	Pyrexia, hyperthyroidism, drugs
Rhythm		
Extra beats (extra systoles)	Rare	Idiopathic
Irregular irregularity	Atrial fibrillation	Drugs
Volume		
Small volume	Aortic or mitral stenosis Cardiac failure	Hypotension

Table 1.11   Features of cardiac disorders

Cardiac disorder	Salient features	Special pre-operative considerations
Congestive cardiac failure	Breathlessness, swollen ankles, on diuretics/digoxin	Consult cardiologist
Ischaemic heart disease	Angina, previous myocardial infarct	Avoid surgery for 3 months after myocardial infarction
Cardiac arrhythmias	Palpitations On cardiac drugs	Consult cardiologist
Valvular lesions	Variable	Antimicrobial cover needed

Table 1.12   Common causes of abnormal blood pressure

Raised	Depressed
Hypertension	Shock
Anxiety	Septicaemia, Addison's disease

Examination of the chest

(1) Inspect the chest wall to exclude vertebral deformities such as side to side curvatures (scoliosis) or anteroposterior curvatures (kyphosis), abnormal chest shape or lesions, and the position of the trachea, which may be abnormal where there is a shift of the mediastinum.

(2) Study respiratory movement. It should be regular, at about 12–14 breaths/minute, with equal movement on both sides of the chest and no obvious exertion either in expiration or inspiration.

(3) Percuss by tapping the mid phalanx of the middle finger of the left hand placed on the chest with the pad of the right middle finger, mainly in order to detect any dullness that signifies abnormal liquid, abnormal tissue or a collapsed lung.

(4) Auscultation with the stethoscope, comparing both lung fields, should elicit any abnormality in quality or quantity of breath sounds, such as wheezing (rhonchi) caused by airways obstruction, crackling sounds (crepitations) caused by liquid in the bronchi or lungs, or a leathery sound (pleural rub) caused by pleural disorders. Voice sounds are normally muffled, but change in quality in some disorders, eg pneumonia (Tables 1.13 to 1.14).

Examination of cranial nerves (Table 1.15)

Urinalysis (Table 1.16)

Table 1.13 Common symptoms and signs of respiratory disease

Symptoms and signs	Respiratory causes	Other causes
Breathlessness (dyspnoea)	Obstructive airways disease	Cardiac disease; anaemia; renal failure
Noisy breathing, wheezing	Bronchial or bronchiolar spasm (eg asthma)	—
Stridor	Laryngeal obstruction	—
Cough	Bronchitis Asthma; carcinoma, bronchiectasis	Cardiac failure
Cyanosis	Severe respiratory disease	Cardiac disease
Rapid breathing (tachypnoea)	Pulmonary fibrosis; emphysema	Intra-abdominal lesions; hysteria; metabolic acidosis
Finger clubbing	Bronchiectasis; carcinoma	Cirrhosis Gastro-intestinal disorders; idiopathic

Table 1.14 Main physical signs in important lung disorders

Signs	Collapse due to obstruction of		Pleural effusion	Pneumothorax	Emphysema	Consolidation (as in lobar pneumonia)
	Major bronchus	Peripheral bronchus				
Chest movement	Reduced on affected side	Reduced on affected side	Reduced or absent on affected side	Reduced or absent on affected side	Symmetrically diminished	Reduced on affected side
Mediastinal displacement	Towards side of lesion	± towards side of lesion	Towards opposite side	Towards opposite side	—	—
Percussion	Dull	Dull	Stony dull	Normal or hyper-resonant	Normal or hyper-resonant over both lungs	Dull
Breath sounds	Reduced or absent	Bronchial	Usually reduced or absent	Usually reduced or absent	Reduced vesicular with prolonged expiration	Bronchial
Voice sounds	Reduced or absent	Increased	Reduced or absent	Reduced or absent	Normal or reduced	Increased
Added sounds	None	None early	± pleural rub	None	Rhonchi and coarse crepitations (from associated bronchitis)	Crepitations

Table 1.15   Examination of cranial nerves

	Nerve	Examination findings in lesions
I	Olfactory	Impaired sense of smell for common odours (do not use ammonia)
II	Optic	Visual acuity reduced using Snellen types ± ophthalmoscopy: nystagmus. Visual fields by confrontation impaired; may be impaired pupil responses
III	Oculomotor	Diplopia; strabismus; eye looks down and laterally; movements impaired; ptosis; pupil dilated. Pupil reactions: direct reflex impaired but consensual reflex intact
IV	Trochlear	Diplopia, particularly on looking down; strabismus; no ptosis; pupil normal and normal reactivity
V	Trigeminal	Reduced sensation over face; ± corneal reflex impaired; ± taste sensation impaired; motor power of masticatory muscles reduced, with weakness on opening jaw; jaw jerk impaired; muscle wasting
VI	Abducens	Diplopia; strabismus; eye movements impaired to affected side
VII	Facial	Impaired motor power of facial muscles on smiling, blowing out cheeks, showing teeth, etc; corneal reflex reduced; ± taste sensation impaired
VIII	Vestibulo-cochlear	Impaired hearing (tuning fork at 256 Hz); impaired balance; ± nystagmus
IX	Glossopharyngeal	Reduced gag reflex; deviation of uvula; reduced taste sensation; voice may have nasal tone
XI	Accessory	Motor power of trapezius and sternomastoid reduced
XII	Hypoglossal	Motor power of tongue impaired, with abnormal speech; ± fasciculation, wasting, ipsilateral deviation on protrusion

1.3 Radiodiagnosis

The x-ray request form

This should be completed and signed by the dentist. It should include:

(1) Vital patient data: full name, address, age, *unit number*, ward or outpatient department or consultant in charge.

Table 1.16 Urinalysis: interpretation of results[a]

	Protein[b]	Glucose[b]	Ketones	Bilirubin[c]	Urobilinogen[c]	Blood[d]
Health	Usually no protein, but a trace can be normal in young people	Usually no glucose, but a trace can be normal in 'renal glycosuria' and pregnancy	Usually no ketones, but ketonuria may occur in vomiting, fasting or starved patients	Usually no bilirubin	Usually present in normal healthy patients, particularly in concentrated urine	Usually no blood
False positives	Alkaline urine. Container contaminated with disinfectant, eg chlorhexidine. Blood or pus in urine. Polyvinyl pyrrolidone infusions	Cephamandole. Container contaminated with hypochlorite	Patients on L-dopa or any phthalein compound	Chlorpromazine and other phenothiazines	Infected urine. Patients taking ascorbic acid, sulphonamides or paraminosalicylate	Menstruation Container contaminated with some detergents
Disease	Renal diseases. Also cardiac failure, diabetes, endocarditis, myeloma, amyloid, some drugs, some chemicals	Diabetes mellitus. Also in pancreatitis, hyperthyroidism, Fanconi syndrome, sometimes after a head injury, other endocrinopathies	Diabetes mellitus. Also in febrile or traumatised patients on low carbohydrate diets	Jaundice. Hepatocellular and obstructive	Jaundice: Haemolytic, hepatocellular and obstructive. Prolonged antibiotic therapy	Genito-urinary diseases. Also in bleeding tendency, some drugs, endocarditis

[a] Using test strips, eg Ames Reagent Strips, BM-Test-5L, Diastix or Diabur strips. Normal or non-fresh urine may be alkaline; normal urine may be acid.
[b] Dopa, ascorbate or salicylates may give false negatives.
[c] May be false negative if urine not fresh.
[d] Ascorbic acid may give false negative.

(2) Details that facilitate correct investigation and accurate opinion:
- investigation required (region to be examined and, where relevant, special investigation needed);
- diagnostic problem;
- relevant clinical features;
- known diagnoses;
- previous relevant operations;
- other information, ie last menstrual period, date, place and type of previous radiographs, whether patient is a walking or trolley case, etc, whether an urgent or routine report is required.

Radiation

Because of the cumulative effect of radiation hazard, all investigations must be justified by benefiting the patient. The clinician requesting the examination or investigation must satisfy himself that it is necessary.

Wherever possible, x-ray investigations on women of child-bearing age should be restricted to the ten days following the start of a menstrual period (the ten-day rule), especially those examinations with a relatively high gonad radiation risk. To facilitate this, a box is provided on the request form for recording the date of the last menstrual period. Note whether the patient is taking the contraceptive pill, has had a hysterectomy, or has been sterilised.

A particular problem arises during pregnancy, because of the hazard to the foetus. The clinician should always ascertain whether a woman is pregnant before requesting a radiograph. All investigations required on pregnant patients should be discussed with the patient and radiologist first.

Portable x-rays

The quality of portable films is rarely as good as that of corresponding films taken in the radiology department.

Examination should take place in the ward, only if there is an absolute contra-indication to the patient being brought to the department. If there is any doubt about the advisability of bringing the patient to the department, consult a radiologist. Theatre radiography is done only when its results are needed during the operation.

Radiography of the mouth

Most dental disorders can be diagnosed clinically, sometimes using intra-oral radiography, although panoramic radiography is particularly useful for showing a wide field and may reveal clinically unsuspected pathology.

Intra-oral radiography

The usual intra-oral views are periapical radiographs, which are useful for demonstrating pathology in the periapical region (abscess, granuloma, cyst) and in the tooth root and adjacent bone, and bitewing radiographs, which show both upper and lower premolar and molar teeth on one film. Bitewings do not show the tooth apex, but are useful in that they reveal approximal caries, and also demonstrate the alveolar crest.

Panoramic radiography

Panoramic radiography is valuable as a general survey, but lacks the detail obtained by periapical radiography. The radiation dose to the patient using panoramic radiography is considerably lower than a full mouth screen using eleven periapical films (Table 1.17), so that a useful compromise is often to take a panoramic view for a general survey, together with two or three intra-oral views of the lesion in question, in order to give detail (Table 1.18). Panoramic radiography does not show detail in the anterior jaws.

Orthodontic radiographs

Orthodontic radiographs are:
(1) Rotated oblique lateral (L and R), nasal–occlusal, or panoramic.
(2) Cephalometric lateral skull. This is obligatory where fixed appliance therapy or orthognathic surgery is a possibility, but is not usually required if the case is amenable to treatment by removable appliances.

Table 1.17   Energy imparted to head and neck (mJ) by different radiographic techniques[a]

Morita Panex E		0·45
SS White Panorex		0·62
GE Panelipse		0·76
Philips Ortho-oralix		1·10
Fiad Rotograph		1·40
Siemens OPG		1·40
Sanki Panograph		4·50
Full mouth periapicals (11)	at 45 kV	3·00
	at 65 kV	4·40
Two bitewings each side	at 45 kV	1·00
	at 65 kV	1·50
One oblique lateral each side		0·40

[a]Adapted from Wall *et al*. *Br J Radiol* 1979; **52:** 727.

Table 1.18 Radiographs recommended for demonstrating lesions at various sites

Radiography requests: To enable the radiographic staff to give you the best or most appropriate radiographs for the region under investigation:

(1) Fill in the request form as fully as possible with full, relevant clinical findings.

(2) Request the region required rather than specific views, except for panoral tomography, when OPT or OPG will suffice

| | Views | |
Region required	Standard	Additional
Skull*	PA 20 Lateral Townes (1/2 axial view)	SMV Tangential
Facial bones	OM OM 30 Lateral	Zygoma Reduced exposure SMV
Paranasal sinuses	OM for maxillary antra	Upper occlusal or lateral SMV OPT, tomography
Orthodontics	OPT/OPG Cephalometric lateral skull	
Pre- and post-osteotomy	OPT/OPG Cephalometric lateral skull Cephalometric PA skull	
Nasal bones	OM 30 Lateral Soft tissue lateral	
Mandible	OPT/OPG	Lateral obliques PA mandible Mandibular occlusal
Temporomandibular joints	Transcranial lateral obliques *or* OPT/OPG (mouth open and closed)	Transpharyngeal Arthrography Reverse Townes Reverse OPT

*CAT scanning is valuable in craniofacial injuries.

Because elective extractions form part of most orthodontic treatment plans, it is extremely important to be systematic in the examination of orthodontic radiographs. Look in order at:

(a) crowns—condition, position, account for *all* teeth;

(b) roots—dilaceration, root resorption;

(c) bone around the roots—evidence of apical or interdental bone loss;

(d) other structures—condyles, antra, etc.

Where canines are thought to be ectopic, localising parallax views may be necessary, ie intra-oral films to compare with the nasal–occlusal.

Fracture radiographs (see Tables 1.18 and 8.4)

1.4 Blood tests

Taking a blood sample (Table 1.19)
(1) Ask a physician to take the sample if
  (*a*) it is a 'renal' patient (their veins are valuable);
  (*b*) the patient usually has difficulty having venepuncture;
  (*c*) you have real doubt as to the success of your venepuncture;
  (*d*) you fail twice to obtain the sample.
(2) Equipment needed to hand before starting:
  (*a*) tourniquet
  (*b*) skin cleansing swab (eg isopropyl alcohol)
  (*c*) gauze swab
  (*d*) syringe
  (*e*) needle (size 19 or 20-gauge for adults, 21 or 23-gauge for children)
  (*f*) containers for sample, labelled with patient's name and number
  (*g*) elastoplast (or alternative adhesive bandage if allergic)

Table 1.19 Complications of venepuncture

Complication	Remarks
Failure in a young normal adult	Relax. Check that the syringe and needle *will* aspirate. Try the other arm; use a sphygmomanometer cuff at just below diastolic pressure; make sure you can palpate the vein before trying again
Difficult patients	
Fat arm: veins difficult to locate	Remember that the veins *are* there. Palpate the antecubital fossa over the usual vein site (see text). If unsuccessful, try the veins on the radial side of the wrist or on the back of the hand (painful)
Thin arm: veins move away from needle	Most annoying! Insert the needle deliberately alongside the vein, preferably at a Y-junction and immobilise the vein with your other hand before penetrating vein from the side
Hepatitis risk patient	See Section 3.9
Haematoma formation	Most annoying to the patient! May cause venous thrombosis. Try not to penetrate through the other side of the vein. Keep gentle pressure with swab on vein after venepuncture until haemostasis secured. In the elderly, maintain this pressure for several minutes

(3) Sites for venepuncture:
- (a) The antecubital fossa. Most commonly used; veins are usually large and easily seen.
- (b) Forearm veins. Venepuncture easy but painful here.
- (c) Veins of the dorsum of the hand. Venepuncture often painful.
- (d) Femoral vein. This vein should be used as a last resort. The artery is midway between the anterior superior iliac spine and the symphysis pubis. The femoral vein is just medial to the femoral artery at the groin.

(4) A 20-gauge needle is the most satisfactory. The needle may be used straight, or bent at a slight angle (especially useful when the syringe is over 20 ml in size or has a central needle fitment).

(5) Clean the skin with a swab. Insert the needle obliquely through the skin in the line of the vein pointing towards the heart. A decrease in resistance is felt when the vein wall is penetrated. Blood is withdrawn slowly, making sure that there is no air in the syringe. Too rapid removal of blood may cause haemolysis.

(6) When sufficient blood has been obtained, release the tourniquet, press swab over the site while the needle and syringe are removed, and hold swab in place with the arm elevated. Always remove the needle before placing blood in specimen tube as this will prevent haemolysis. Great care should be taken to avoid spillage of blood and to avoid needle pricks. Remove the tourniquet as soon as possible and also roll down the sleeve, which can otherwise continue to act as a tourniquet.

(7) Gently introduce blood into the correct container. If the specimen tube contains anticoagulant, ensure mixing by gently rolling the capped tube.

(8) Carefully dispose of the needle in the sharps container.

(9) Label the tube with the patient's name, number, date and time, etc.

(10) Complete and sign the appropriate request form and give relevant clinical data, patient's name and number, etc.

Precautions

- Make sure the tourniquet is not too tight or else the arterial supply and venous return will both be decreased. Blood samples for platelet counts and blood calcium estimation require that the tourniquet should be loosened after insertion of the needle and before taking blood.
- If the patient is on a drip, take blood samples from the arm that does not have the drip.
- Always use the correct bottle for the correct test and do not allow the blood to haemolyse by keeping it too long.

- Muscle pump. This is a very useful technique to aid distention of veins, but it can significantly increase the serum potassium level and it should not be used unless absolutely necessary.
- For jaundiced patients, or those with HB_sAg or HIV (see Section 3.9).

1.5 Histology and cytology

Surgical specimens and biopsies for histology and immunology
Complete the request form and give a clinical résumé, the dates, and the serial numbers, of all previous biopsies.

Histology
Put small specimens immediately into buffered formalin solution in at least its own volume of fixative. Put large specimens into fixative in plastic bags. Leave formalin-fixed specimens at room temperature. Potentially

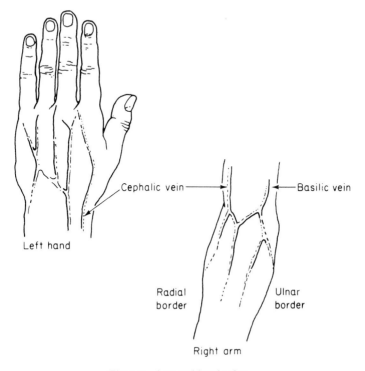

Fig. 1.3 Arm and hand veins.

infectious tissues (eg tuberculous) should be placed in formalin immediately, but if bacteriological examination is required, send a separate specimen without fixative.

Immunology
Specimens are not usually fixed, but immediately snap-frozen (on solid CO_2 or liquid nitrogen).

Biopsy technique

Mucosa or skin
Include some normal tissue as well as the lesion (biopsies of ulcers alone are inadequate). Do not squeeze with forceps. Sutures may be used to hold the tissue and also to mark specific areas of the biopsy. Place tissue on to a small piece of paper before immersing in fixative, to prevent curling.

Lymph node
Lymph nodes have a blood supply which must be ligated before excision. Lymph nodes are often closely related to large veins and sometimes large arteries. Some lymph nodes are closely related to important nerves. Some pathologists like to make an imprint from the fresh cut surface of lymph nodes. They may wish to do this personally. Make an adequate skin incision. Do not squeeze node or fragment it, but remove it whole. Put it straight into fixative, unless some is needed for culture or guinea pig inoculation.

Labial salivary gland
Make a linear mucosal incision (lower labial mucosa). Excise at least four lobules of salivary gland.

Frozen sections for rapid diagnosis
Communicate with the pathologist at the latest by the day before the operation. Telephone the laboratory when the specimen is on its way. Warn the pathologist about any tissue containing calcified material *before* he breaks his microtome.

Oral smears for cytology
Take smears with a wooden or metal spatula, or dental plastic instrument. Spread evenly on the centres of two previously labelled glass slides and fix immediately in industrial methylated spirit. Do not allow to dry in air, as cellular detail is rapidly lost and artefacts develop. After 20 minutes of

fixation, the smears can be left to dry in the air or left in fixative; in this way, smears will keep for up to three weeks.

1.6 Microbiology and immunology

Bacterial infections
Collect all specimens for microbiology fresh from the patient and send them to the laboratory. Specify any chemotherapy on the request form. Most microbiological examinations require at least overnight incubation of cultures. In particularly urgent situations, or where anaerobes may be present, discuss the case with a microbiologist.

Antibiotic sensitivity tests
In most cases, the bacteria must first be isolated and cultured before their sensitivity may be tested, but direct sensitivity tests are sometimes of value. In urgent cases, ask for immediate sensitivity tests.

Isolates are tested against a number of antibacterial agents which are relevant to the organism in question, but are not all necessarily suitable to the particular infection present. The best choice must be made on clinical and other grounds.

Antibiotic assays
Assays are most commonly required during treatment with aminoglyco-sides (gentamicin, streptomycin, kanamycin, tobramycin), to ensure that adequate, but non-toxic, serum concentrations are reached.

Usually, two specimens are required, each of 5 ml of clotted blood, one taken within the hour before a dose of aminoglycoside, and the other taken after a dose (one hour after if by intramuscular route, 5 minutes after if by intravenous route, when the sample should be from a different site from the injection).

Pus
Avoid contamination from the surrounding mucosa or skin when taking swabs from wounds or abscesses. Whenever possible, send actual pus collected in a syringe or dry sterile bottle rather than a swab. Certain agents, such as actinomyces, can rarely be detected in the small amount of pus available on a swab. If there is any likelihood of delay in specimens reaching the laboratory, swabs should be placed in a transport medium and pus refrigerated at 4–8°C (a normal refrigerator). The source of the pus or swab must be indicated clearly; for example, the site of the wound should

be stated. Any particular pathogen suspected should also be mentioned, so that the most relevant techniques may be used.

Antral washings
Use sterile saline and send fresh to the laboratory in sterile containers.

Blood cultures
If bacteraemia or septicaemia is suspected, three or more cultures are needed. If bacterial endocarditis is suspected, cultures are usually required on two or more consecutive days, but if it is considered desirable to start treatment earlier, more than one culture may be taken on the same day. It is rarely necessary to take more than three cultures, unless the patient has recently received antibiotics.

Procedure
(1) Disinfect the skin with two applications of 0·5% chlorhexidine in 70% alcohol, or two impregnated swabs, allowing at least a minute for the disinfectant to act before inserting the needle.
(2) Collect 10 ml blood with a clean venepuncture.
(3) Change the needle on the syringe, taking care not to contaminate the nozzle of the syringe.
(4) Remove the cellophane wrap from each of two culture bottles (one for aerobic, one for anaerobic, culture) and inject 5 ml blood into each bottle.
(5) Do not swab the cap of the bottles with disinfectant.
(6) Send the bottles at once to the laboratory, with a request form; if there is no urgency, out of hours, the bottles should be placed in a 37°C incubator provided for blood cultures.

Exudates and transudates
Ten to twenty millilitres should be put into a sterile universal container, except where tuberculosis is suspected, when a large amount should be sent in two sterile 100-ml bottles with citrate to prevent clotting.

Serological tests
For all serological investigations, 10 ml clotted blood in a dry, sterile (white-capped; see Tables 1.20 and 1.21) bottle is required and should reach the laboratory within 24 hours. Serological tests for syphilis are shown in Table 3.18. Serological tests for many uncommon infections (ie parasitic infections) are available from Reference Laboratories. Consult a microbiologist. Before HIV testing, counselling is required.

Sputum

Deliver sputum expectorated directly into the special containers provided, as far as possible uncontaminated by saliva, fresh to the laboratory. State the type of infection suspected.

Nasal swabs

Collect nasal discharge with a swab and treat as pus. Detect staphylococcal carriers by swabbing both anterior nares with the same swab, moistened with sterile saline. The swab should be rotated to procure as large a sample as possible.

Oral and pharyngeal swabs

Swabs must be well rubbed over the fauces, particularly the tonsillar area and any membrane if present. If diphtheria is suspected, this should be mentioned.

Candida infection of the mouth and pharynx (thrush) is best determined by examination of a Gram smear made at the bedside, from a spatula firmly scraped across a lesion. The presence of hyphal forms suggests a pathogenic role for the *Candida*. A swab should also be sent for culture.

Tissues

Biopsy specimens, etc, for culture should be sent in dry, sterile containers. Formalin must not be added.

Urine

Detection of urinary tract infection depends on the assessment of numbers of bacteria present; normal urine should not contain more than 10 000 bacteria/ml (usually much fewer) which are contaminants from the urethra and skin. Infected urine generally has more than 100 000/ml. The nature of the bacteria isolated may be important; commensals (such as lactobacilli) are of no significance.

For these criteria to hold, urine must be cleanly collected and examined when fresh, usually collected after a small amount of urine has been passed (mid-stream urine, MSU). The urine must be received in the laboratory within two hours of being passed. Urinary organisms multiply at room temperature and cells may undergo lysis. If further delay is inevitable, the urine must be refrigerated at 4°C. If neither of these courses is possible, a dip inoculum technique may be used. A special slide bearing culture medium obtained from the laboratory is dipped into the urine as soon as it has been passed into a sterile vessel. The excess is drained off, and the slide

Table 1.20 Interpretation of haematological results

Blood	Normal range[a]	Level ↑	Level ↓	Comments on collection[b]
Haemoglobin	Male 13·0–18·0 g/dl Female 11·5–16·5 g/dl	Polycythaemia (vera or physiological) myeloproliferative disease	Anaemia	EDTA tube (pink top)
Haematocrit (packed cell volume or PCV)	Male 40–54%; female 37–47%	Polycythaemia; dehydration	Anaemia	EDTA tube (pink top)
Mean cell volume (MCV)	78–99 fl; $MCV = \dfrac{PCV}{RBC}$	Macrocytosis in vitamin B12 or folate deficiency; liver disease; alcoholism; hypothyroidism; myelodysplasia; myeloproliferative disorders; aplastic anaemia; cytotoxic agents	Microcytosis in iron deficiency; thalassaemia; chronic disease	EDTA tube (pink top)
Mean cell haemoglobin (MCH)	27–31 pg; $MCH = \dfrac{Hb}{RBC}$	Pernicious anaemia	Iron deficiency; thalassaemia; sideroblastic anaemia	EDTA tube (pink top)
Mean cell haemoglobin concentration (MCHC)	32–36 g/dl; $MCHC = \dfrac{Hb}{PCV}$		Iron deficiency; thalassaemia; sideroblastic anaemia; anaemia in chronic disease	EDTA tube (pink top)
Red cell count (RBC)	Male 4·2–6·1 $\times 10^{12}$/litre; female 4·2–5·4 $\times 10^{12}$/litre	Polycythaemia	Anaemia; fluid overload	EDTA tube (pink top)
White cell count Total	4–10 $\times 10^{9}$/litre	Pregnancy; exercise; infection; trauma; leukaemia	Early leukaemia; some infections; bone marrow disease; drugs; idiopathic	EDTA tube (pink top)

Table 1.20 Interpretation of haematological results—*contd*

Blood	Normal range[a]	Level ↑	Level ↓	Comments on collection[b]
Neutrophils	average 3×10^9/litre	Pregnancy; exercise; infection; bleeding; trauma; malignancy; leukaemia	Some infections; drugs; endocrinopathies; bone marrow disease; idiopathic	EDTA tube (pink top)
Lymphocytes	average 2·5 $\times 10^9$/litre	Physiological; some infections; leukaemia; bowel disease	Some infections; some immune defects (eg AIDS)	EDTA tube (pink top)
Eosinophils	average 0·15 $\times 10^9$/litre	Allergic disease; parasitic infestations; skin disease; lymphoma	Some immune defects	EDTA tube (pink top)
Platelets	150–400 $\times 10^9$/litre	Thrombocytosis in bleeding; myeloproliferative disease	Thrombocytopenia related to leukaemia; drugs; infections; idiopathic; autoimmune	EDTA tube (pink top)
Reticulocytes	0·5–1·5% of RBC	Haemolytic states; during treatment of anaemia	—	EDTA tube (pink top)
Erythrocyte sedimentation rate (ESR)	0–15 mm/hour	Pregnancy; infections; anaemia; connective tissue disease; myelomatosis; malignancy; temporal arteritis	—	Citrated tube (black top)
Plasma viscosity	1·4–1·8 cp	As ESR	—	EDTA tube (pink top). Relative viscosity of plasma cf. water

[a] Adults unless otherwise stated. Check values with your laboratory.
[b] Vacuum tubes differ in colour; Vacutainer(s) are: EDTA tube (pink top); citrated tube (black top).
MCH: mean corpuscular haemoglobin; MCHC: mean corpuscular haemoglobin concentration.

Table 1.21 Interpretation of biochemical results

Biochemistry[a]	Normal range[b]	Level ↑	Level ↓	Comments on collection[c]
Acid phosphatase	0–13 IU/litre	Prostatic malignancy; renal disease; acute myeloid leukaemia	—	White top tube. Separate serum immediately. Haemolysed blood unsuitable
Alanine transaminase (ALT)[d]	3–60 IU/litre	Liver disease; infectious mononucleosis	—	White top tube
Alkaline phosphatase	30–110 IU/litre (3–13 KA units)	Puberty; pregnancy; Paget's disease; osteomalacia; fibrous dysplasia; malignancy in bone, liver disease; hyperparathyroidism (some); hyperphosphatasia	Hypothyroidism; hypophosphatasia; malnutrition	White top tube
Alpha-1-antitrypsin	200–400 mg%	Cirrhosis	Congenital emphysema	White top tube
Alphafoetoprotein	<12 μg/litre	Pregnancy; gonadal tumour; liver disease	Drop in pregnancy indicates foetal distress	White top tube
Amylase	70–300 IU/litre	Pancreatic disease; mumps; some other salivary diseases	—	White top tube
Antistreptolysin 0 titre (ASOT)	0–300 Todd units/ml	Streptococcal infections; rheumatic fever	—	White top tube
Aspartate transaminase (AST)[e]	3–40 IU/litre	Liver disease; biliary disease; myocardial infarct; trauma	—	White top tube
Bilirubin (total)	1–17 μmol/litre	Liver or biliary disease; haemolysis	—	White top tube
Caeruloplasmin	1·3–3·0 μmol/litre	Pregnancy; cirrhosis; hyperthyroidism; leukaemia	Wilson's disease	White top tube

Table 1.21 Interpretation of biochemical results—*contd*

Biochemistry[a]	Normal range[b]	Level ↑	Level ↓	Comments on collection[c]
Calcium	2·3–2·6 mmol/litre (*Total* calcium)	Hyperparathyroidism (some); malignancy in bone; renal tubular acidosis; sarcoidosis; thiazides	Hypoparathyroidism; renal failure; rickets; nephrotic syndrome	White top tube. Collect with tourniquet off. Repeat several times for reliability. Assay albumin as well
Cholesterol	3·9–7·8 mmol/litre	Hypercholesterolaemia; pregnancy; hypothyroidism; diabetes; nephrotic syndrome; liver or biliary disease	Malnutrition; hyperthyroidism	White top tube. Collect fasting sample
Complement (C3)	0·79–1·60 g/litre	Trauma; surgery; infection	Liver disease; immune complex diseases: eg lupus erythematosus	—
(C4)	0·2–0·4 g/litre	—	Liver disease; immune complex diseases; HANE	—
Cortisol (see steroids)				
Creatine phosphokinase (CPK)	50–100 IU/litre (<130)	Myocardial infarct; trauma; muscle diseases	—	White top tube. Serum must be separated immediately
Creatinine	0·06–0·11 mmol/litre	Renal failure; urinary obstruction	Pregnancy	White top tube
C reactive protein (CRP)	<10 mcg/ml	Inflammation; trauma; myocardial infarct; malignant disease	—	White top tube
C1 esterase inhibitor	0·1–0·3 g/litre	—	Hereditary angioedema	White top tube

Table 1.21 Interpretation of biochemical results—*contd*

Biochemistry[a]	Normal range[b]	Level ↑	Level ↓	Comments on collection[c]
Ferritin	Adult male 25–190 ng/ml Adult female 15–99 ng/ml Child mean 21 ng/ml	Liver disease; haemochromatosis; leukaemia; lymphoma; other malignancies; thalassaemia	Iron deficiency	White top tube. Better than assay of serum iron
Fibrinogen	200–400 mg%	Pulmonary embolism; nephrotic syndrome; lymphoma	Disseminated intravascular coagulopathy (DIC)	White top tube
Folic acid	3–20 µg/litre (red cell folate 120–650 µg/litre)	Folic acid therapy	Alcoholism; dietary deficiency; haemolytic anaemias; malabsorption; myelodysplasia; phenytoin; methotrexate; trimethoprim; pyrimethamine; sulphasalazine; cycloserine; oral contraceptive	EDTA tube (pink top)
Free thyroxine index (FTI) (serum T4 × T3 uptake)	1·3–5·1 U	Hyperthyroidism	Hypothyroidism	White top tube
Gammaglutamyl transpeptidase (GGT)	(5–42 IU/litre)	Liver disease; myocardial infarct; pancreatitis, diabetes; renal diseases; tricyclics	—	White top tube
Globulins (total) (see also under protein)	22–36 g/litre	Liver disease; myelomatosis; autoimmune disease; chronic infections	Chronic lymphatic leukaemia; malnutrition; protein-losing states	White top tube

Table 1.21 Interpretation of biochemical results—*contd*

Biochemistry[a]	Normal range[b]	Level ↑	Level ↓	Comments on collection[c]
Glucose	2·8–5·0 mmol/litre	Diabetes mellitus; pancreatitis; hyperthyroidism; hyperpituitarism; Cushing's disease; liver disease; after head injury	Hypoglycaemic drugs; Addison's disease; hypopituitarism; hyperinsulinism; severe liver disease	Collect fasting or at least 2 hours after meal: special fluoride bottle (yellow top)
Hydroxybutyrate dehydrogenase (HBD)	100–250 IU/litre	Myocardial infarct	—	White top tube
Immunoglobulins Total	7–22	Liver disease; infection; sarcoidosis; connective tissue disease	Immunodeficiency; nephrotic syndrome; enteropathy	White top tube
IgG	5–16 g/litre	Myelomatosis; connective tissue diseases	Immunodeficiency; nephrotic syndrome	White top tube
IgA	1·25–4·25 g/litre	Alcoholic cirrhosis; Buerger's disease	Immunodeficiency	White top tube
IgM	0·5–1·75 g/litre	Primary biliary cirrhosis; nephrotic syndrome; parasites; infections	Immunodeficiency	White top tube
IgE	<0·007 mg%	Allergies; parasites	—	White top tube
Lactic dehydrogenase (LDH)	90–300 IU/litre	Myocardial infarct; trauma; liver disease; haemolytic anaemias; lymphoproliferative diseases	Radiotherapy	White top tube. Unsuitable if blood haemolysed
Lipase	0·2–1·5 IU/litre	Pancreatic disease	—	White top tube
Lipids	50–150 mg% (triglycerides)	Hyperlipidaemia; diabetes mellitus; hypothyroidism	—	White top tube. Collect fasting sample

Table 1.21 Interpretation of biochemical results—*contd*

Biochemistry[a]	Normal range[b]	Level ↑	Level ↓	Comments on collection[c]
Magnesium	0·7–0·9 mmol/litre	Renal failure	Cirrhosis; malabsorption; diuretics; Conn's syndrome; renal tubular defects	White top tube
Nucleotidase	1–15 IU/litre	Liver disease	—	White top tube
Phosphate	0·8–1·5 mmol/litre	Renal failure; bone disease; hypoparathyroidism; hypervitaminosis D	Hyperparathyroidism; rickets; malabsorption syndrome; insulin	White top tube. Collect fasting sample. Separate serum promptly
Potassium	3·5–5·0 mmol/litre	Renal failure; Addison's disease	Vomiting; diabetes; diarrhoea; Conn's syndrome; diuretics; Cushing's disease; malabsorption	White top tube. Fresh blood should be sent to laboratory. Haemolysis causes abnormal results
Protein (total)	62–80 g/litre	Liver disease; myelomatosis sarcoid; connective tissue diseases	Nephrotic syndrome; lymphomas; enteropathy; renal failure	White top tube. Collect fasting sample
Albumin	35–55 g/litre	Dehydration	Liver disease; malabsorption; nephrotic syndrome; myelomatosis; connective tissue disorders	White top tube
Alpha 1 globulin	2–4 g/litre	Oestrogens	Nephrotic syndrome	White top tube
Alpha 2 globulin	4–8 g/litre	Infections; trauma	Nephrotic syndrome	White top tube
Beta globulin	6–10 g/litre	Hypercholesterolaemia; liver disease; pregnancy	Chronic disease	White top tube
Gamma globulin	6–15 g/litre	(see Immunoglobulins)	Nephrotic syndrome; immunodeficiency	White top tube

Table 1.21 Interpretation of biochemical results—*contd*

Biochemistry[a]	Normal range[b]	Level ↑	Level ↓	Comments on collection[c]
SGGT (see GGT) SGOT (see AST) SGPT (see ALT)				
Sodium	130–145 mmol/litre	Dehydration; Cushing's disease	Oedema; renal failure; Addison's disease	White top tube
Steroids (corticosteroids)	110–525 nmol/litre ($14 \pm 6 \mu g\%$)	Cushing's disease; some tumours	Addison's disease; hypopituitarism	White top tube. Collect at 08.00–09.00 hours
Thyroxine (T4)	50–138 nmol/litre	Hyperthyroidism; pregnancy; contraceptive pill	Hypothyroidism; nephrotic syndrome; phenytoin	White top tube
Urea	3·3–6·7 mmol/litre	Renal failure; dehydration	Liver disease; nephrotic syndrome; pregnancy	White top tube
Uric acid	0·15–0·48 mmol/litre	Gout; leukaemia; renal failure; myelomatosis	Liver disease; probenecid; allopurinol; salicylates; other drugs	White top tube. Serum must be separated immediately
Vitamin B12	150–800 ng/litre	Liver disease; leukaemia	Pernicious anaemia; gastrectomy; Crohn's disease; ileal resection; vegans	White top tube

Note: Values may differ from laboratory to laboratory. For further information, consult R. D. Eastham. *Biochemical values in clinical medicine.* Bristol: Wright, 1975. There are many more causes of abnormal results than are outlined here.

[a] Serum or plasma

[b] Adult levels; always consult your own laboratory

[c] Vacuum tubes differ in colour – for 'white top' read 'brown top' and for 'yellow top' read 'grey top'

[d] ALT = SGPT (serum glutamate-pyruvate transaminase).

[e] AST = SGOT (serum glutamate-oxaloacetic transaminase)

SI values: $10^{-1} = $ deci (d); $10^{-2} = $ centi (c); $10^{-3} = $ milli (m); $10^{-6} = $ micro (μ); $10^{-9} = $ nano (n); $10^{-12} = $ pico (p); $10^{-15} = $ femto (f).

is returned to its container and sent to the laboratory with the urine specimen.

The mode of collection of the urine (mid-stream, clean, or catheter specimen), the date and time of collection, and any chemotherapy, must be stated on the request form. For tubercle bacilli, three early morning urines (EMU, complete specimen rather than mid-stream) are required.

Table 1.22 Significance of the more common antinuclear antibodies

Antinuclear antibodies	Associated with	Significance
Diffuse (homogeneous)	Antibodies to deoxyribo-nucleoprotein	High titres: SLE Low titres: other connective tissue diseases
Rim (peripheral)	Antibody to double stranded DNA (DS-DNA)	Antibody with the highest specificity for SLE and found in most patients
Speckled	Antibodies to extractable nuclear antigens (ENA)	to Smith (Sm) antigen: very specific for SLE but only seen in minority of cases to Ribonuclear protein (nRNP or UIRNP) antigen: mixed connective tissue disorder, scleroderma, SLE to Robert (Ro) soluble substance A antigen (SS-A): SLE skin disease: some Sjögren's syndrome to Lane (La) soluble substance B antigen (SS-B): SLE and primary and secondary Sjögren's syndrome JO-1: polydermatomyositis PM-SC1[a]: polydermatomyositis, and scleroderma to Centromere: Crest syndrome
Nucleolar	Antibodies to nucleolus specific RNA	Scleroderma
DNA antibodies	DS-DNA (*Crithidia luciliae*)	High titres: SLE
	SS-DNA	Rheumatic diseases and chronic inflammatory disorders (not specific but sensitive)

Key: SS-DNA = single stranded DNA; DS-DNA = double stranded DNA; SLE = systemic lupus erythematosus; CREST = calcinosis, Raynaud's, oesophageal, sclerodactyly and telangiectasia.
[a] SC1-70 = anti-topoisomerase 1.

Table 1.23 Other autoantibodies that may be useful in diagnosis in dentistry*

Autoantibody	Significance	Remarks[a]
Rheumatoid factor[b]	Latex test > 1 in 20 SCAT > 1 in 32 DAT > 1 in 16	May imply RA (sometimes SLE)
Other Salivary duct antibody		Positive in Sjögren's syndrome, particularly in Sicca syndrome

Parietal cell antibody;
  intrinsic factor
  antibodies
		Positive in pernicious anaemia

Epithelial intercellular cement		Positive in pemphigus
Epithelial basement membrane zone		Positive in some pemphigoid

[a] See Appendix for abbreviations
[b] Agglutination tests. SCAT = sheep cell agglutination test; DAT = direct agglutination test.
*The presence of autoantibodies does not always indicate disease

Viral infections
Virological testing is costly.

Virus isolation
Send all specimens without delay to the laboratory. If no transport is available, swabs may be stored in viral transport medium for a few hours at 4°C. Use sterile swabs with wooden sticks and then immediately break off into a bottle of virus transport medium. Vesicle fluid, urine, faeces, cerebrospinal fluid, biopsies and post-mortem material should be put into a sterile container.

Serology
Serum for investigation for markers of hepatitis or HIV should be collected and handled with special precautions (see Section 3.9).

For serological tests, sterile clotted blood should reach the laboratory within 24 hours, or the serum should be separated and stored frozen at − 20°C. It is important to take two specimens of blood, the first (acute serum) as early as possible in the illness and the second (convalescent serum) ten or more days later. A fourfold rise in antibody titre is indicative of infection.

Electron microscopy
Vesicle fluid (or crusts if this cannot be obtained) can be examined for the
rapid diagnosis of herpes simplex and diagnosis of varicella/zoster or orf.

Autoantibody investigations
The mere presence of autoantibodies, particularly if they are in low titre,
does *not* necessarily signify disease. See Tables 1.22 and 1.23 for interpretation of autoantibody results, bearing the above comment in mind.

1.7 Records and confidentiality

Good clear and accurate records are essential to good practice and patient
care and, increasingly, are important medicolegally. Clear and reasonably
frequent communication with the referring clinician/primary care physician or dentist is essential, not only to ensure care of the patient but also to
maintain and enhance professional relationships.

Records should be:
- in ink or type, not pencil;
- legible;
- dated;
- signed clearly (with your name in capitals if the signature is obscure);
- factually accurate (take especial care on tooth notation);
- complete.

Records should not:
- be subsequently altered unless the alteration is signed and dated, as in
  the case of an altered bank cheque;
- contain confusing abbreviations or acronyms;
- contain obscene, sarcastic or other unprofessional comments.

Correspondence with referring and other clinicians
Apart from patient details, this should contain:
- the name of the responsible clinician or consultant;
- the date the patient was seen;
- the history, diagnosis, clinical course, treatment and prognosis;
- any information of which the patient should or should not be informed.

Confidentiality
Information about a patient is sometimes requested by a 'third party'.
Unless you have written permission from the person in question to divulge

the information, to do so is an invasion of privacy and is unethical. However, common sense should prevail and clearly the spouse should, for example, normally receive information as to post-operative progress, etc. On the other hand, such details should never be disclosed to others, such as the press or media.

The following are guidelines, but always elicit the policy of your seniors and the institute in which you work.

(1) *Always* identify the inquirer.

(2) It is *always* best to check with the patient if information can be imparted and to whom.

(3) Do *not* give information to members of the press or media, or the police, without checking with your seniors (indeed, the wise person avoids *any* contact with the media!).

(4) Try and give any information to relatives in person whenever possible and not over the telephone. Do not delegate the task.

Access to Medical Reports Act 1988

This UK Act of Parliament gives patients right of access to their health reports, and permits them to request the clinician to make alterations if they feel the contents are inaccurate.

Data Protection Act 1984

This UK Act grants access to computer-held records.

Medicolegal reports

Such reports should only be prepared with the express consent of the patient or his solicitor.

(1) Give the patient's full surname and first name, date of birth, address and occupation.

(2) State the reason for the report.

(3) Make it clear who was the responsible clinician for the clinical care related to the incident involved.

(4) Give the date, time and place, if the report is from a specific examination of the patient.

(5) Clearly and accurately summarise the history given by the patient and the history as shown by the clinical records.

(6) Clearly and accurately summarise the examination findings and results of investigations.

(7) Clearly and accurately summarise the treatment given.

(8) Clearly and accurately summarise the clinical course and prognosis.

Remember that this may involve legal proceedings.

2
Oral Diseases

An ABC of symptoms and signs of oral diseases

Anaesthesia
See paraesthesia and sensory loss.

Blisters
True blisters (see Table 2.1)
Skin diseases
    *Pemphigoid (usually mucous
      membrane pemphigoid)
    Pemphigus
    Erythema multiforme
    Dermatitis herpetiformis/Linear IgA
      disease
    Epidermolysis bullosa
    Lichen planus (very rarely)

Infections
    Herpes simplex
    Herpes zoster-varicella

Others
    Burns
    Angina bullosa haemorrhagica

False blisters
Cysts
Mucoceles
Abscesses

Burning mouth
Psychogenic
    *Cancerophobia
    Depression
    Anxiety states
    Hypochondriasis

Deficiency states
    Vitamin B12 deficiency
    Folate deficiency
    Iron deficiency

Infections
    Candidosis

Others
    Erythema migrans (geographical
      tongue)
    Diabetes
    Captopril

Cacoguesia (unpleasant taste in the mouth)
Oral infections
    Chronic periodontitis
    Acute ulcerative gingivitis
    Chronic dental abscesses
    Dry socket
    Pericoronitis

Xerostomia
    Drugs
    Sjögren's syndrome
    Irradiation damage

Psychogenic causes
    Depression
    Anxiety states
    Psychoses
    Hypochondriasis

Drugs (see Table 5.21)

Starvation

*Most common cause.

Cacoguesia—contd
Nasal disease
  Chronic sinusitis
  Oro-antral fistula

Gastric regurgitation

Frontal lobe tumours

Liver disease

Discharges
Dental disease
  *Chronic dental abscess
  Pericoronitis
  Dry socket
  Cysts
  Oro-antral fistula
  Osteomyelitis
  Osteoradionecrosis

Salivary gland disorders
  Sialadenitis

Psychogenic
  Depression
  Hypochondriasis

Psychosis

Dry mouth
Drugs with anticholinergic effects
  Atropine and analogues
  Tricyclic antidepressants
  Antihistamines
  Anti-emetics
  Phenothiazines
  Antihypertensives

Drugs with sympathomimetic actions
  Decongestants
  Bronchodilators
  Appetite suppressants
  Amphetamines

Dehydration
  Uncontrolled diabetes mellitus
  Diabetes insipidus
  Diarrhoea and vomiting
  Severe haemorrhage

Psychogenic
  Anxiety states

Depression
Hypochondriasis

Salivary gland disease
  Sjögren's syndrome
  Irradiation damage
  Sarcoidosis
  HIV
  Ectodermal dysplasia

Dysarthria
Oral disease
  *Painful lesions (or loss of mobility,
    particularly of the tongue or
    palate)
  Cleft palate

Neurological disorders
  Multiple sclerosis
  Parkinsonism
  Cerebrovascular accident
  Bulbar palsy
  Hypoglossal nerve palsy
  Cerebral palsy
  Myopathies

Drugs
  Alcohol
  Phenothiazines
  Levodopa
  Butyrophenones

Severe xerostomia

Dysphagia
Oral disease
  *Inflammatory, traumatic, surgical
    or neoplastic lesions of tongue,
    palate or pharynx

Xerostomia

Oesophageal disease
  Foreign bodies
  Stricture
  Carcinoma
  Systemic sclerosis

Pharyngeal pouch

Psychogenic
  Hysteria

Neurological disorders
  Stroke
  Bulbar palsy
  Syringobulbia
  Achalasia
  Myopathies

Facial palsy
Neurological disease
  *Bell's palsy
  Stroke
  Cerebral tumour
  Moebius syndrome
  Multiple sclerosis
  Trauma to facial nerve or its
    branches
  Leprosy
  Ramsay-Hunt syndrome
  Guillain-Barré syndrome

Middle ear disease
  Cholesteatoma
  Mastoiditis

Parotid
  Parotid cancer

Others
  Melkersson-Rosenthal syndrome
  Sarcoidosis (Heerfordt syndrome)
  Myopathies
  Lyme disease
  HIV

Facial swelling
(Facial swelling is commonly
    inflammatory in origin, caused by
    cutaneous or dental infection or
    trauma)

Inflammatory
  *Oral infections
  Cutaneous infections
  Insect bites

Traumatic
  Post-operative oedema or
    haematoma
  Traumatic oedema or haematoma
  Surgical emphysema

Immunological
  Allergic angioedema
  Hereditary angioedema

Endocrine and metabolic
  Systemic corticosteroid therapy
  Cushing syndrome
  Myxoedema
  Acromegaly
  Obesity
  Nephrotic syndrome

Superior vena cava syndrome
    (obstruction to SVC, eg by
    bronchial carcinoma)

Cysts

Neoplasms

Foreign body

Others
  Crohn's disease
  Melkersson-Rosenthal syndrome
  Congenital (eg lymphangioma)

Halitosis
Oral infections
  *Chronic periodontitis
  Infections
  Acute ulcerative gingivitis
  Dry socket
  Oral abscesses
  Nasal infections and foreign bodies

Xerostomia

Foods
  Garlic
  Curries
  Onions

Drugs
  Solvent abuse
  Alcohol
  Chloral hydrate
  Nitrites and nitrates
  Dimethyl sulphoxide
  Cytotoxic drugs
  Phenothiazines
  Amphetamines
  Smoking

Halitosis—*contd*
Systemic disease
  Respiratory tract infections
  Cirrhosis
  Liver failure
  Renal failure
  Diabetic ketosis
  Gastrointestinal disease
  Psychogenic

Hyperpigmentation

Generalised
*Racial

Food/drugs

Endocrinopathies
  Addison's disease
  Nelson's syndrome
  Inappropriate ACTH production

Others
  Albright syndrome
  Haemochromatosis
  Drugs (see Table 5.21)
  ACTH therapy

Localised
  *Amalgam tattoo
  Ephelis
  Pigmentary incontinence
  Melanoma
  Naevus
  Peutz-Jegher syndrome
  Kaposi's sarcoma

Loss of taste

Anosmia
  *Upper respiratory tract infections
  Maxillofacial fracture

Neurological disease
  Cerebrovascular disease
  Multiple sclerosis
  Bell's palsy
  Fractured base of skull
  Posterior cranial fossa tumours
  Cerebral metastases

Psychogenic
  Anxiety states
  Depression
  Psychoses

Drugs
  Penicillamine

Irradiation

Xerostomia

Zinc or copper deficiency

Pain (see also Fig. 2.1; Table 2.2)

Local diseases
Diseases of the teeth and supporting
    tissues
  *Pulpitis
  Periapical periodontitis
  Lateral (periodontal) abscess
  Acute ulcerative gingivitis
  Pericoronitis

Diseases of the jaws
  Dry socket
  Fractures
  Osteomyelitis
  Infected cysts
  Malignant neoplasms

Diseases of the maxillary antrum
  Acute sinusitis
  Malignant neoplasms

Diseases of the salivary glands
  Acute sialadenitis
  Calculi or other obstruction to duct
  Severe Sjögren's syndrome
  Malignant neoplasms

Diseases of the eyes
  Glaucoma

Vascular disorders
Migraine

Migrainous neuralgia

Temporal arteritis (giant cell arteritis)

Neurological disorders
Trigeminal neuralgia
Malignant neoplasms involving the
  trigeminal nerve
Multiple sclerosis
Bell's palsy (occasionally)
Herpes zoster (including
  post-herpetic neuralgia)

Psychogenic pain
Atypical facial pain and other oral
  symptoms associated with anxiety
  or depression, eg mandibular
  pain–dysfunction

Referred pain
Angina
Lesions in the neck or chest
  (including lung cancer)

Paraesthesia and sensory loss
Peripheral causes
  *Surgical damage to nerves
    (including local analgesic
    injections)
  Fractures of the jaws
  Osteomyelitis
  Pressure by a lower denture on the
    mental nerve
  Neoplasms in antrum or
    nasopharynx
  Tumour deposits in mandible or
    pterygomandibular space

Intracranial disease
  Multiple sclerosis
  Tumours
  Syringobulbia
  Surgical treatment of trigeminal
    neuralgia
  Cerebrovascular disease

Psychogenic
  Hyperventilation syndrome
  Hysteria

Drugs (see Table 5.21)
  Acetozolamide
  Labetalol
  Sulthiame

Benign trigeminal sensory neuropathy

Tetany

Some connective tissue diseases

Hysteria

Pigmentation see Hyperpigmentation

Purpura
*Trauma

Platelet and vascular disorders
  Thrombocytopenia (especially drugs
    and leukaemias)
  Thrombasthenia
  Von Willebrand's disease
  Scurvy
  Ehlers-Danlos syndrome
  Chronic renal failure

Infections
  Infectious mononucleosis
  Rubella
  HIV
  Amyloidosis

Red areas
Localised red patches
  *Denture stomatitis
  Erythroplasia
  Purpura
  Telangiectases
  Angiomas (purple)
  Chemical burns
  Lichen planus
  Lupus erythematosus
  Kaposi's sarcoma

Generalised redness
  *Candidosis
  Avitaminosis B (rarely)
  Irradiation mucositis
  Mucosal atrophy
  Polycythaemia

Sialorrhoea

Painful lesions or foreign bodies (for example new dentures) in the mouth may cause increased salivation, as may cholinergic drugs (as used in myasthenia gravis), buprenorphine and, rarely, rabies. The term sialorrhoea may be given to drooling of saliva as a result of poor neuromuscular coordination, as in infants, the mentally handicapped, Parkinsonism or facial palsy.

Trismus

Extra-articular causes
  Infection and inflammation near
    masticatory muscles
  Mandibular pain–dysfunction
    syndrome
  Fractured condylar neck
  Fibrosis (including systemic
    sclerosis and submucous fibrosis)
  Tetanus
  Tetany
  Invading neoplasm
  Myositis ossificans
  Coronoid hypertrophy or fusion to
    zygomatic arch
  Hysteria

Intra-articular causes
  Dislocation
  Intracapsular fracture
  Arthritides
  Ankylosis

Ulcers

Local causes
*Traumatic
  (may be artefactual)

Chemical, electrical, thermal, radiation

Neoplastic
Carcinoma and other tumours

Recurrent aphthous stomatitis
  (including Behçet's and Sweet's
  syndromes)

Ulcers associated with systemic disease
Cutaneous disease
  Erosive lichen planus
  Pemphigus
  Pemphigoid
  Erythema multiforme
  Dermatitis herpetiformis/Linear IgA
    disease

Blood disorders
  Anaemia
  Neutropenia
  Leukaemia

Gastrointestinal
  Coeliac disease
  Crohn's disease
  Ulcerative colitis

Connective tissue disease
  Lupus erythematosus

Reiter's disease

Infective
  Herpetic stomatitis
  Chickenpox
  Herpes zoster
  Hand, foot and mouth disease
  Herpangina
  Infectious mononucleosis
  HIV
  Acute ulcerative gingivitis
  Tuberculosis
  Syphilis
  Histoplasmosis or blastomycosis
    (rarely)

Drugs (especially cytotoxics)

Others

White patches

Developmental
  White sponge naevus
  Other rare syndromes

Acquired

Persistent white lesions
   *Frictional
   Smoker's keratosis
   Syphilitic keratosis
   Idiopathic keratosis
   Chronic candidosis
   Lichen planus
   Lupus erythematosus
   Dysplastic (dyskeratotic) lesions
   Verrucous carcinoma
   Early invasive carcinoma
   Skin grafts
   Chronic renal failure
   Hairy leukoplakia (HIV)
   Some papillomas

Transient white lesions
   Chemical burns
   Thrush
   Cheek biting

Xerostomia see **Dry mouth**

The antrum
Discharge from nose
Sinusitis (usually acute)

Foreign body

Malignant disease

Pain
Sinusitis
   Acute sinusitis
   Chronic sinusitis

Malignant disease
   Squamous carcinoma
   Other neoplasms

Fungal infections (rarely)

Swelling
Fibro-osseous lesion

Malignant disease

The gingiva
Red areas
Redness of the gums is common and usually a sign of chronic gingivitis but is then restricted to the gingival margins. More generalised redness is a sign of 'desquamative gingivitis', usually caused by lichen planus or mucous membrane pemphigoid (see also **Swelling**).

Bleeding
Periodontal disease
   *Chronic gingivitis
   Chronic periodontitis
   Acute ulcerative gingivitis

Haemorrhagic diseases
   Platelet and vascular disorders
   Leukaemia
   HIV
   Idiopathic thrombocytopenic purpura
   Hereditary haemorrhagic
     telangiectasia
   Ehlers-Danlos syndrome
   Scurvy
   Angiomas

Drugs
   Anticoagulants
   Aspirin
   Cytotoxics
   Sodium valproate

Clotting defects
   Liver disease
   Obstructive jaundice
   Haemophilia
   von Willebrand's disease

Swelling
Generalised gingival swelling
   *Chronic 'hyperplastic' gingivitis
   Drug-induced (phenytoin,
     cyclosporin, nifedipine, diltiazem)
   Hereditary gingival fibromatosis
   Leukaemia
   Mucopolysaccharidosis
   Mucolipidosis
   Wegener's granulomatosis
   Scurvy

Swelling—*contd*
Localised gingival swellings
  *Abscesses
  Cysts
  Pyogenic granulomas
  Neoplasms (including fibrous epulis)
  Giant cell lesions
  Foreign bodies
  Wegener's granulomatosis
  Sarcoidosis
  Amyloidosis

Ulcers

Ulcers that affect predominantly the gingivae are usually traumatic, acute ulcerative gingivitis or occasionally result from immunodeficiency—especially acute leukaemia, HIV or agranulocytosis. The gingivae can, however, be affected by most other causes of mouth ulcers.

The lips

Angular stomatitis (cheilitis)
Candidosis
Staphylococcal, streptococcal or mixed infections
Ariboflavinosis (rarely), iron, folate or B12 deficiency
Crohn's disease
Anaemia
HIV

Bleeding
*Trauma
Cracked lips
Acute erythema multiforme
Angiomas

Underlying haemorrhagic disease inevitably aggravates any tendency to bleed from labial lesions.

Blisters
*Herpes labialis
Burns
Herpes zoster
Erythema multiforme
Pemphigus vulgaris
Mucoceles
Impetigo

Desquamation and crusting
Dehydration, particularly exposure to hot dry winds
Chemical or allergic cheilitis
Erythema multiforme
Psychogenic

Swellings
There is a wide individual and racial variation in the size of the lips

Diffuse swellings
  Oedema (trauma or infection or insect bite)
  Angioedema: allergic or hereditary
  Crohn's disease
  Cheilitis granulomatosa
  Cheilitis glandularis
  Melkersson-Rosenthal syndrome
  Lymphangioma
  Haemangioma

Localised swellings
  Mucoceles
  Chancre
  Tumours
    Salivary adenoma
    Squamous cell carcinoma
    Other tumours
    Keratoacanthoma
  Cysts
  Abscesses
  Insect bite

Ulceration
Trauma
Infective
  Herpes labialis
  Herpes zoster
  Syphilis
  Aphthae (occasionally)

Tumours
  Squamous cell carcinoma

Burns

Lupus erythematosus

White lesions
*Keratoses
Carcinoma
Lichen planus
Lupus erythematosus
Fordyce's spots
Actinic keratosis
Scars

The neck
Swellings in the neck

Cervical lymph nodes
  *Lymphadenitis (pharyngeal, dental,
    tonsillar, face or scalp infections)
  Infectious mononucleosis
  Tuberculosis or other mycobacterial
    infections
  Secondary carcinoma (oral,
    nasopharyngeal or thyroid
    primary)
  Lymphoma
  Leukaemia
  Acquired immune deficiency
    syndrome (+ persistent
    lymphadenopathy syndrome)
  Other infections (cat scratch disease,
    staphylococcal, syphilis,
    toxoplasmosis)

Other
  Connective tissue diseases,
  sarcoid, mucocutaneous lymph
  node syndrome (Kawasaki disease)

Salivary gland
  *Mumps
  Tumours
  Sjögren's syndrome
  Sarcoidosis
  Sialadenitis

Side of the neck
  Actinomycosis
  Branchial cyst
  Parapharyngeal cellulitis
  Pharyngeal pouch
  Cystic hygroma
  Carotid tumours

Mid-line of the neck
  Thyroglossal cyst
  Thyroid tumours or goitre
  Deep ranula
  Ludwig's angina
  Dermoid cyst

The palate
Lumps
Developmental
  *Unerupted teeth
  Torus palatinus
  Cysts

Inflammatory
  Abscesses
  Cysts
  Necrotising sialometaplasia

Neoplasms
  Oral or antral carcinoma
  Salivary tumours
  Fibrous overgrowths
  Kaposi's sarcoma
  Papillomas
  Others
  Foreign bodies

Redness
Redness restricted to the denture-bearing
area of the palate is almost invariably denture
stomatitis (candidosis). Other red lesions
may be erythroplasia

The salivary glands
Swellings
Inflammatory
  *Mumps
  Sjögren's syndrome
  Ascending sialadenitis
  Recurrent sialadenitis
  Sarcoidosis
  Actinomycosis

Neoplasms
  Benign (pleomorphic adenoma;
    adenolymphoma or Warthin's
    tumour, adenoma, oxyphil
    adenoma)

The salivary glands—*contd*
Swelling—*contd*
Neoplasms—*contd*
  Malignant (malignant PSA, adenoid
    cystic carcinoma, adenocarcinoma,
    mucoepidermoid carcinoma, acinic
    cell carcinoma, squamous
    carcinoma)

Others
  *Duct obstruction
  Sialosis
  Mikulicz disease (lymphoepithelial
    lesion and syndrome)

Drug-associated
  Chlorhexidine
  Phenylbutazone
  Iodine compounds
  Thiouracil
  Catecholamines
  Sulphonamides
  Phenothiazines
  Methyldopa

Salivary gland pain

Common causes
  *Mumps
  Stones or other causes of
    obstruction

Rare causes
  Sjögren's syndrome
  Acute sialadenitis
  Recurrent sialadenitis
  Salivary gland malignant tumours

Drug-associated
  Antihypertensive drugs
  Cytotoxic drugs
  Vinca alkaloids

The temporomandibular joint
Ankylosis

Trauma
Infection
Inflammatory (juvenile RA, ankylosing
  spondylitis, RA)

Dislocation

Trauma
Phenothiazines (rarely)
Hysteria (rarely)

Limitation of opening of jaw
(see **Trismus**)
Usually muscle spasm secondary to
  local inflammation

Pain

Mandibular pain-dysfunction
  syndrome
Inflammation
Infection
Penetrating injury
Haematogenous, eg gonococcus

Non-infective causes
  Traumatic arthritis
  Rheumatoid arthritis
  Osteoarthrosis
  Gout
  Psoriatic arthropathy

Neoplasms
  Benign
  Malignant (primary or metastases)

The tongue
Swellings or lumps

Localised
Congenital
  Lingual thyroid
  Hamartomas

Inflammatory
  Post-operative infection
  Insect bite

Traumatic
  Oedema
  Haematoma

Neoplastic
  *Fibrous lump
  Papilloma
  Carcinoma
  Granular cell tumour

Others
    Foreign body
    Cyst

Diffuse
Congenital
    Down's syndrome
    Cretinism
    Mucopolysaccharidoses

Inflammatory
    Post-operative infection
    Insect bite

Traumatic
    Oedema
    Haematoma

Neoplastic
    Lymphangioma
    Haemangioma

Others
    Multiple endocrine adenomatosis
        type III
    Angioedema
    Amyloidosis
    Cyst
    Acromegaly

Sore tongue

With obvious lesions
    Any cause of oral ulceration (see
        above)
    *Geographical tongue
    Median rhomboid glossitis

Glossitis (generalised redness and
    depapillation)

Anaemia
Candidosis (rarely)
Avitaminosis B (very rarely)
Post-irradiation

With no physical abnormality
Anaemia
Depression or cancerophobia

Oral complaints that are frequently or invariably psychogenic

It is essential to exclude organic causes for the following:

Dry mouth
Sore or burning mouth
Bad taste or disturbed taste
Atypical facial pain
Atypical odontalgia
Paraesthesias and anaesthesia
Mandibular pain–dysfunction
    syndrome
Non-existent discharges
'Gripping' dentures
Vomiting or nausea caused by
    dentures
Supposed sialorrhoea
Non-existent lumps
Multiple complaints (the 'syndrome of
    oral complaints')

Disorders of the teeth (see Table 2.3)

Table 2.1 Differentiation of the more common vesiculobullous disorders

	Pemphigus	Benign mucous membrane pemphigoid	Erythema multiforme	Dermatitis herpetiformis[d]	Lichen planus[c]	Angina bullosa haemorrhagica
Incidence	Rare	Uncommon	Uncommon	Rare	Uncommon	Common
Age mainly affected	Middle age	Late middle age	Young adults	Middle age	Middle age	Middle age
Sex mainly affected	F	F	M	M	F	F
Geographic factors	Italians, Jews	—	—	—	—	—
Predisposing factors	—	—	Drugs; infections	Gluten	Drugs	—
Oral manifestations	Erosions; blisters rarely persist; Nikolsky sign positive	Blisters (sometimes blood-filled); erosions; Nikolsky sign may be positive	Swollen lips; serosanguinous exudate; large erosions anteriorly; occasional blisters	Blisters; ulcers	White lesions; erosions; rarely bullae	Blood-filled blisters often on soft palate
Cutaneous manifestations	Large flaccid blisters sooner or later	Rare or minor	Target or iris lesions may be present	Pruritic vesicular rash on back and extensor surfaces	Pruritic, papular on flexor surfaces	—
Histopathology	Acantholysis; intra-epithelial bulla	Subepithelial bulla	Subepithelial bulla	Subepithelial bulla	Hyperkeratosis; acanthosis; basal cell liquefaction	Subepithelial bulla
Direct immunofluorescence	Intercellular IgG in epithelium	Subepithelial/ BMZ[a]; C3; IgG	Subepithelial IgG[b]	Subepithelial IgA	Variably IgM/fibrin C3[b] at BMZ[a]	—
Serology	Antibodies to epithelial intercellular cement in most	Antibodies to epithelial basement membrane in few	—	Antibodies to reticulin in some	—	—
Other investigations or features	—	—	—	Biopsy of small intestine	—	—

[a] BMZ = basement membrane zone.
[b] Non-specific findings.
[c] Rarely bullous.
[d] And linear IgA disease.

Table 2.2   Differentiation of important types of facial pain[a]

	Idiopathic trigeminal neuralgia	Atypical facial pain	Migraine	Migrainous neuralgia
Age (years)	> 50	30–50	Any	30–50
Sex	F > M	F > M	F > M	M > F
Site	Unilateral, mandible or maxilla	± Bilateral, maxilla	Any	Retro-orbital
Associated features	—	± Depression	± Photophobia; ± nausea; ± vomiting	± Conjunctival infection; ± lacrimation; ± nasal congestion
Character	Lancinating	Dull	Throbbing	Boring
Duration of episode	Brief (seconds)	Continual	Many hours (usually day)	Few hours (usually night)
Precipitating factors	± Trigger areas	None	± Foods ± stress	Alcohol ± stress
Relieving factors	Carbamazepine	Antidepressants	Clonidine; ergot derivatives	Clonidine; ergot derivatives

[a] Most oral pain is caused by local disease.

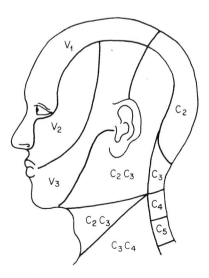

Fig. 2.1   Sensory nerve supply to the head and neck.

Table 2.3 Disorders of the teeth

Symptom or sign	Teeth usually affected	Most common causes	Less common causes	Least common causes
Late eruption	Any	Genetic variance; impacted teeth	Hypopituitarism; hypothyroidism; cleidocranial dysplasia	Various genetic disorders; irradiation; cytotoxic drugs
Missing teeth	Third molars; lateral incisors; second premolars	Genetic variance; impacted teeth; extracted teeth	Ectodermal dysplasia; cleidocranial dysplasia; Down's syndrome	Various genetic disorders
Extra teeth	Usually anteriorly, often in maxilla	Genetic variance; supernumerary; retention of deciduous precursors	Cleidocranial dysplasia; predeciduous dentition (natal teeth)	Various genetic disorders
Malpositioned teeth	Canines; second premolars	Crowding; supernumeraries	Abnormal muscle action (eg cerebral palsy); cleft palate	Scarring; various genetic disorders
Malformed teeth	Second premolars; maxillary incisors	Infected precursor (Turner teeth); trauma to developing tooth	Intra-uterine infections; genetic variance	Various genetic disorders; irradiation; cytotoxic drugs
Discoloured teeth	Any; often the maxillary incisors	Extrinsic stain (drugs, smoking); caries; trauma (dead tooth); root treatment	Tetracycline; fluorosis; osteogenesis imperfecta; amelogenesis imperfecta; dentinogenesis imperfecta	Kernicterus; porphyria
Painful teeth	Any	Caries (pulpitis)	Trauma: abrasion, erosion, attrition	Irradiation; trigeminal herpes zoster; neoplasms
Premature loosening of teeth	Any	Exfoliating primary teeth; chronic periodontal disease	Trauma	Neoplasms; juvenile periodontitis; other forms of severe periodontitis hypophosphatasia; Ehlers-Danlos syndrome; hyperthyroidism; histiocytosis; Papillon-Lefevre syndrome

3

Systemic Diseases of Particular Importance in Dentistry

The medical history should be directed to elicit any systematic disease relevant to dentistry. For example:

A: Anaemia   F: Fits and faints (Chapter 4)
B: Bleeding tendency   G: Genito-urinary and other infections
C: Cardiac   H: Hepatitis and liver disease
D: Drugs and drug abuse   I: Important other conditions,
E: Endocrine disease   eg pregnancy

3.1 Anaemia

Anaemia is a reduction in haemoglobin level below the normal for age and sex. It can (*a*) be a contra-indication to general anaesthesia; (*b*) cause oral complications, ie sore mouth, burning tongue, glossitis, ulcers, angular stomatitis. Anaemia is caused mainly by reduced erythropoiesis, haemolysis, or haemorrhage. The most usual cause of anaemia in the UK is iron deficiency caused by chronic haemorrhage (commonly menorrhagia).

Investigation of anaemia

After a thorough history and examination, a full blood film, red cell indices, haemoglobin concentration and white cell count and differential are required for diagnosis of the extent and type of anaemia (Table 3.1). The cause must then be established.

Deficiency anaemias

Once the type of anaemia has been established (Tables 3.1, 3.2), the cause must be found and treated. In iron deficiency, unless it is clear that menorrhagia is the cause, the site of blood loss should be sought, usually in the gastrointestinal tract.

Iron deficiency anaemia is treated by (*a*) treatment of the cause, (*b*) iron supplements (Table 3.3). Only rarely is transfusion necessary, usually when the haemoglobin is less than 9 g/dl and operation is required urgently. Packed red cells should be used in preference to blood (see Section 7.10).

Table 3.1 Investigations of iron deficiency and iron deficiency anaemia[a]

	MCV	Hb	MCH or MCHC[b]	Serum ferritin	Transferrin saturation (%)[c]	Marrow iron stores
Normal	N	N	N	N	33	N
Mild iron deficiency anaemia	↓	N or ↓	N	↓	> 16	↓
Moderate iron deficiency anaemia	↓	↓	↓	↓	< 16	↓
Severe iron deficiency anaemia	↓↓	↓↓	↓↓	↓↓	< 16	↓

[a] See Table 1.20 for abbreviations
Arrows indicate a value below normal (N).
Note: It is now preferable to measure serum ferritin levels if this assay is available, as it is more indicative of low iron stores than is the transferrin saturation.
[b] The MCH is preferable if automatic Coulter assay is used.
[c] Transferrin saturation = serum iron concentration/total iron binding capacity.

Table 3.2 Anaemias in which there are changes in iron status

Type of anaemia	Serum ferritin levels	Serum iron levels	TIBC[a]	Marrow iron	Sideroblasts present
Iron deficiency	↓	↓	↑	↓	Nil
Thalassaemia	↑	N or ↑	N or ↑	N or ↑	N or ↑
Chronic disease	↓	N or ↓	N or ↓	↑	Nil
Sideroblastic	↑	↑	↓	↑↑	↑↑

[a] Total iron-binding capacity.

Table 3.3 Treatment of iron deficiency

Preparation	Trade name (example)	Adult oral dose[a]
Ferrous sulphate	Many examples: use Ferrous Sulphate tablets BNF	1 tablet, 2 or 3 times a day
Ferrous fumarate	Fersaday	1 tablet (304 mg), 1 or 2 times a day
Ferrous glycine	Ferrocontin continus	1 tablet (563 mg), 1 daily

[a] Take with meals and continue therapy for a further 6 months after haemoglobin has returned to normal level.

Table 3.4   Drugs used in megaloblastic anaemias

Drug	Comments	Adult dose
Folic acid	Indicated in folate deficiency but not in B12 deficiency, as it may precipitate neurological damage	5 mg, up to 4 times orally a day (usually once a day)
Vitamin B12 (hydroxocobalamin injection)	Needed for the rest of patient's life	1000 μg every 1 to 3 months IM
Folinic acid	Used in patients on methotrexate and other folate antagonists to reduce oral ulceration (Leucovorin 'rescue')	120 mg divided over 12 hours IM or IV then 15 mg orally every six hours

Folate deficiency is commonly dietary in origin. Treatment is outlined in Table 3.4.

Vitamin B12 deficiency is rarely dietary in origin; more commonly it is caused by a gastrointestinal lesion or pernicious anaemia. Prolonged exposure to nitrous oxide may result in vitamin B12 inhibition. Treatment is outlined in Table 3.4.

Deficiencies of multiple factors, eg iron, folate and vitamin B12, may well be caused by disease of the small intestine.

Sickle cell anaemia
Sickle cell anaemia is a hereditary condition affecting haemoglobin, found mainly in black patients and some originating from the Mediterranean countries and Asia.

Homozygous form: sickle cell anaemia
In these patients, at low oxygen tensions (about 45 mmHg), the red cells become inelastic and sickle shaped; they then either 'sludge', blocking capillaries and causing infarcts (eg in marrow and brain), or rupture, causing haemolytic anaemia. General anaesthesia may be dangerous to these patients and should not be given in a dental practice.

Heterozygous form: sickle cell 'trait'
In patients with the sickle trait, sickling occurs only at much lower oxygen tensions (below 20 mmHg), which are unlikely to occur in normal clinical practice.

Diagnosis

(1) Check the medical history.
(2) Screen all black patients. Do a full blood picture and a screening test, and record results in the patient's notes. Also record negative results, to prevent unnecessary retesting.

A simple solubility test (eg the SickleDex test) will detect the presence of any HbS in the blood and is therefore positive both in patients with sickle cell anaemia and the trait. Further haematological examination, including haemoglobin electrophoresis, is theoretically required for confirmation. In practice, however, a positive solubility test with a normal haemoglobin level can be taken as being diagnostic of the trait, anaemia being inevitable in homozygotes.

Management

Sickle cell anaemia
Even mild deprivation of oxygen can prove fatal in patients with sickle cell anaemia. They must be given a general anaesthetic only under 'ideal' conditions, in hospital, by a specialist anaesthetist and usually after a pre-operative blood transfusion. Avoid low body temperature under general anaesthesia, and vasoconstrictors in local anaesthesia. Small local infarcts may result from vasoconstriction and stasis in the immediate area. Treat infections aggressively, as they may precipitate a crisis.

Sickle cell trait
Provided they have a normal haemoglobin level, patients with the trait may be safely treated as outpatients, using either general or local anaesthesia. Care must of course be taken to avoid hypoxia in these patients, but only extreme anoxia is likely to produce sickling and its consequences. Consult a physician first.

3.2 Bleeding tendency

Local causes
Local causes include 90% of post-extraction haemorrhages.● Excessive
● Excessive trauma (to soft tissue in particular).   lar).
● Inflamed mucosa at the extraction site.
● Post-extraction interference with the socket, eg sucking and tongue pushing.
● Reactive hyperaemia.

Management

Press firmly with a moist gauze pad over the socket for 10–15 minutes. If the patient is re-attending, mattress suture the socket under local anaesthetic (±oxidised cellulose or a calcium alginate preparation into the socket). Sedate the anxious patient (5 mg diazepam orally for adults). See Section 7.10 for indications for blood transfusion (rarely needed).

Systemic causes

Defects may be (a) acquired deficiencies of haemostasis, eg anticoagulant therapy, thrombocytopenia, leukaemia; (b) hereditary deficiencies of clotting factors, eg haemophilia.

Significant histories suggesting a bleeding tendency (see also Tables 3.5, 3.6)

- Previous bleeding for more than 36 hours or bleeding restarting more than 36 hours after operation, particularly if on more than one occasion.
- Previous admission to hospital to arrest bleeding.
- Previous blood transfusions for bleeding.
- Spontaneous bleeding, eg haemarthrosis, deep bruising, or menorrhagia from little obvious cause.
- A convincing family history of one of the above, combined with a degree of personal history.
- Recent therapy by significant drugs (anticoagulants or, occasionally, aspirin).

The patient may have a card indicating a bleeding tendency.

Table 3.5   Laboratory findings in clotting disorders

	PT	APTT KPTT	TT	FL	FDP
Haemophilia A (classic haemophilia), Haemophilia B (Christmas disease), deficiency of Factors XI, XII	N	↑	N	N	N
Coumarin therapy, Warfarin therapy, obstructive jaundice, or other causes of vitamin K deficiency, deficiency of Factor V or X	↑	↑	N	N	N
Heparin therapy	↑	↑	↑	N	N
Disseminated intravascular coagulation, parenchymal liver disease	↑	↑	↑	↓	↑
Deficiency of Factor VII	↑	N	N	N	N

PT = prothrombin time; APTT = activated partial thromboplastin time; TT = thrombin time; FL = fibrinogen level; FDP = fibrin degradation products; KPTT = kaolin partial thromboplastin time. Arrows indicate a value above ↑ or below ↓ normal (N).

Table 3.6 Outline of management of haemophiliacs[a] requiring dental surgical procedures

Operation	Factor VIII level required (% of normal)	Immediately pre-operatively give	Post-operative schedule
Minor oral surgery[b]	Minimum of 50% at operation (preferably 75–80%)	Factor VIII, IV[c]; tranexamic acid 1 g, IV (or by mouth starting 24 hours pre-operatively)	Rest in-patient for 7 days unless resident close to centre (then 3 days as in-patient). Soft diet. For 10 days give tranexamic acid 1–1·5 g and penicillin V 250 mg orally every 6 hours. If there is bleeding during this period, give repeat dose of Factor VIII[c]
Maxillofacial surgery	100% at operation; 50% for 7 days post-operatively	Factor VIII, IV[d]	Rest in-patient for 10 days. Soft diet. Twice daily IV Factor VIII[c] for 7–10 days. Penicillin V 250 mg orally every 6 hours

[a] Haemophilia A.
Haemophiliacs should be treated in hospital, preferably in one with a Haemophilia Centre.
[b] In *very* mild haemophilia, 4–6 µg desmopressin IV, at 24 hours pre-operatively, may reduce the amount of Factor VIII or tranexamic acid needed.
[c] Factor VIII dose in units = weight in kg × 25.
[d] Factor VIII dose in units = weight in kg × 50.

Laboratory investigations

Screening tests (mainly platelet count and function tests, APTT, PT and clotting factor assays; Table 3.5) will eliminate two-thirds of the suspected cases, and the remaining third will require more detailed tests to accurately define a diagnosis. Consult the haematologist immediately before undertaking any laboratory investigations; bleeding and clotting times are quite unsatisfactory, and special investigations may well be required, such as factor VIII clotting activity or related antigen assay.

Management in systemic causes: acquired deficiencies

Oral anticoagulant treatment

The WHO and the International Committee for Standardisation in Haematology have recommended that prothrombin times should, in future, be reported as international normalised ratio (INR) The INR is the ratio of the patient's one stage prothrombin time to that of controls. A normal healthy patient has an INR of 1. The following are therapeutic ranges.

	INR range
Deep vein thrombosis prophylaxis	1·5–2·5
Deep vein thrombosis prophylaxis in surgery	2·0–3·0

Anticoagulant therapy will not prevent successful haemostasis using local measures for minor oral surgery, such as the relatively atraumatic removal of one or two teeth, unless the INR is greater than about 2·0 to 2·5 (prothrombin time over 2·0 to 2·5 times normal; prothrombin index below 40%; thrombotest below about 15%). Check the prothrombin time 5–7 days pre-operatively. Adjusting the dose of anticoagulant to give an INR of 1·5–2·0 may be necessary if the INR is much higher, but the responsible haematologist should always be consulted about this. It may be necessary to reduce the warfarin 5–6 days before surgery, but this is indicated mainly if more major surgery is contemplated. Treatment to reverse anticoagulant therapy completely is usually unnecessary and undesirable, since it might cause rebound hypercoagulability.

Always consider the implications of the underlying reason for which the patient is on anticoagulants (eg cardiac prosthesis).

Liver disease (see Section 3.9)

Platelet defects

Thrombocytopenia is significant if platelets are below 80×10^9 per litre. Appropriate measures to raise the platelet count (platelet infusions) are

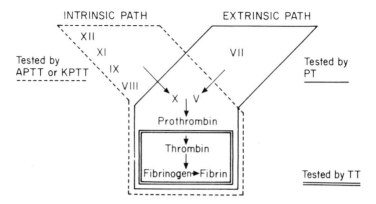

Figure 3.1 The blood clotting cascade. APTT: activated partial thromboplastin time; KPTT: kaolin partial thromboplastin time (= kaolin cephalin clotting time or KCCT); PT: prothrombin time; TT: thrombin time.

required, to allow local measures to succeed. Leukaemia may be associated with thrombocytopenia and anaemia; antifibrinolytic therapy and platelets are appropriate corrective measures, in addition to local treatment.

For further discussion about dental care of patients with leukaemia, see Section 3.11 and the Appendix 6.

Management in systemic causes: hereditary deficiencies

These are mainly clotting defects, corrected by therapy using an appropriate blood product particularly rich in the deficient factor: Factor VIII or cryoprecipitate for haemophilia A and von Willebrand's disease, and Factor IX for Christmas disease (see Fig. 3.1). It has been found, however, that in mild haemophilia A and in von Willebrand's disease, blood products may be used in lower doses if desmopressin (1-deamino-8-D-arginine vasopressin) and antifibrinolytic therapy (epsilon aminocaproic acid or tranexamic acid) are used. Table 3.6 gives further details. Remember that viral hepatitis and AIDS (see Sections 3.8, 3.9) should be considered.

Things to avoid in patients with a bleeding tendency

(see Table 3.7)

- Trauma.
- Regional local anaesthetic injections (may bleed into fascial spaces of neck and obstruct airway).
- Intramuscular injections.
- Drugs causing gastric bleeding (eg aspirin and NSAIDS).
- Drugs causing increased bleeding tendency (eg aspirin).

Table 3.7 Prescribing for patients on warfarin therapy[a]

Type	Avoid	Alternative, if essential
Analgesics	Aspirin/NSAIDS Dextropropoxyphene Mefenamic acid	Paracetamol, codeine
Antibiotics	Sulphonamides (including co-trimoxazole) erythromycin metronidazole tetracyclines	Penicillins, cephalosporins, gentamicin
Hypnotics/ sedatives	Barbiturates	Benzodiazepines
Anti- convulsants	Sodium valproate	Carbamazepine Phenytoin
Others	Alcohol Cimetidine Corticosteroids	

[a]The contraceptive pill reduces the anticoagulant effect.

3.3 Cardiac disease

Points to remember

- Cardiac disease is common.
- Patients with cardiac disease may become breathless if laid flat (as in the dental chair).
- There is no evidence that the adrenaline in local anaesthetic solutions is a hazard to cardiac patients. Indeed, much more endogenous adrenaline is released if the dental procedure is painful (for example where LA without a vasoconstrictor is used). It is more important to ensure adequate anaesthesia but, if you are concerned, it is reasonable to use prilocaine plus felypressin (see Section 6.1).
- A mild premedicant such as 5 mg diazepam orally can be valuable in cardiac patients.
- General anaesthesia constitutes a risk; consult a physician (see Section 6.1). GA is contra-indicated within 3 months of a myocardial infarct and possibly up to 2 years afterwards.
- Cardiac patients may need antimicrobial cover (Section 3.3) or may have a bleeding tendency because of anticoagulants (Section 3.2).

Things to avoid in cardiac patients

- Hypoxia due to poor ventilation.
- Hypotension, by drugs.

- Fluid overload, by IV fluids.
- Respiratory depression, by sedatives; local anaesthesia is preferred to general anaesthesia.
- Anxiety.

Infective endocarditis

Patients with various cardiac lesions are predisposed to develop endocarditis, which may be precipitated as a consequence of the bacteraemia associated with some forms of dental treatment.

Cardiac lesions that predispose to infective endocarditis include congenital cardiac defects, rheumatic heart disease (chorea or St Vitus' dance may predispose), prosthetic cardiac valves, previous history of endocarditis, hypertrophic cardiomyopathy, aortic valve disease (bicuspid valves). Those with a prosthetic cardiac valve, or with a history of endocarditis are at special risk.

Prevention depends on giving prophylactic antimicrobials before dental treatment, particularly tooth extraction, oral surgery, scaling and periodontal surgery. Antimicrobial prophylaxis should be started only a few hours pre-operatively (Table 3.8). A pre-operative mouthwash with aqueous chlorhexidine 0·2% may also be useful.

It is essential to warn patients at risk to report back if even a minor febrile illness develops after dental treatment. Remember that the cardiac lesion may make the patient a poor risk for general anaesthesia, and that those patients with prosthetic valves, may be on anticoagulants and have a consequent bleeding tendency.

3.4   Drugs and drug abuse

Corticosteroids

- Corticosteroids absorbed systemically produce adrenocortical suppression, such that patients cannot respond adequately to the stress of trauma, operation or infection. The suppression may persist for months or years after the steroid treatment (see Chapter 4). Stress may produce collapse in adrenal crisis.
- Injected and oral corticosteroids are most potent at causing adrenocortical suppression, but inhalers or skin creams can occasionally act in the same way.
- Courses of systemic steroid treatment as brief as one week may interfere with adrenocortical responses.
- Patients on steroids, or recently on steroids, usually need steroid supplementation before dental operations (Table 3.9).

Table 3.8   Antimicrobial prophylaxis against infective endocarditis[a]

Local anaesthesia		General anaesthesia		
Not allergic to penicillin	Allergic to penicillin	No other special risk	Special risk, eg previous endocarditis, prosthetic valve	
		Not allergic to penicillin	Not allergic to penicillin	Allergic to penicillin
Amoxycillin	Erythromycin stearate	Amoxycillin	Amoxycillin + gentamicin	Vancomycin + gentamicin
Oral 3 g	Oral 1·5 g then 0·5 g orally after 6 hours	IM 1 g then 0·5 g orally after 6 hours *or* oral 3 g 4 h pre-opera-tively + 1 g probenecid	IM amoxycillin 1 g plus gentamicin 120 mg IM then amoxycillin 0·5 g orally after 6 hours	IV vancomycin 1 g plus gentamicin 120 mg

[a]Start 1 hour pre-operatively unless otherwise stated.

- Patients on steroids should carry a blue warning card to this effect.
- Patients on systemic corticosteroids are also liable to other serious complications, including diabetes, hypertension, psychoses, osteoporosis, and liability to infections (they are immunosuppressed). In children there is growth retardation.

Investigation of adrenocortical function

- Blood pressure.
- Diurnal rhythm of plasma cortisol is a sensitive index of adrenal function; plasma cortisol values are normally highest between 6.0 and 10.0 am and lowest between midnight and 4.0 am. Samples taken at 8.0 am and 4.0 pm should differ by at least 5 μg/100 ml. The sample taken at 8.0 am should be 5–25 μg/100 ml.
- Synacthen test (ACTH stimulation test):
  - (*a*) take 5 ml blood at 8.0 to 9.0 am for plasma cortisol level;
  - (*b*) give 0·25 mg Synacthen subcutaneously or intramuscularly;
  - (*c*) after 30 minutes, take a further blood sample for plasma cortisol level.
- Plain abdominal radiograph.
- Autoantibody titres.
- Electrolytes.

Table 3.9 Suggested management of dental surgery patients with a history of systemic corticosteroid therapy*

	No steroids for previous 12 months	Steroids taken during previous 12 months	Steroids currently taken
Minor surgery (eg single extraction under LA)	No cover required	Give hydrocortisone 200 mg orally[a], IM[b] or IV[b]	Give hydrocortisone 200 mg orally[a], IM[b] or IV[b] pre-operatively. Continue normal steroid medication post-operatively
Intermediate surgery (eg multiple extractions or surgery under GA)[d]	Consider cover if large doses of steroid were given. Test adrenocortical function (ACTH stimulation test)[c]	Give hydrocortisone[b] 200 mg IV pre-operatively and IM 6-hourly for 24 hours	Give hydrocortisone[b] 200 mg IV pre-operatively and IM 6-hourly for 24 hours; then continue normal medication
Major surgery or trauma (eg maxillofacial surgery)[d]	Consider cover if large doses of steroid were given. Test adrenocortical function (ACTH stimulation test)[c]	Give hydrocortisone[b] 200 mg IV pre-operatively and IM 6-hourly for 72 hours	Give hydrocortisone[b] 200 mg IV pre-operatively and IM 6-hourly for 72 hours; then continue normal medication

*Restorative dentistry is not an indication for steroid cover, but monitor BP.
[a] Hydrocortisone given orally 2 hours pre-operatively *or* double the dose of oral steroid the night before and on day of operation.
[b] Hydrocortisone sodium succinate (eg Ef-Cortelan soluble) or phosphate (eg Ef cortesol) given 30 minutes pre-operatively; or 250 mg methyl prednisolone IV.
[c] See Section 3.4.
[d] Monitor blood pressure half-hourly for at least 2 hours if a GA has been given.

Interpretation

- Blood pressure is low in hypoadrenocorticism, high in hyperadrenocorticism.
- Plasma cortisol at 8.0 to 9.0 am is often below $6 \, \mu g/100 \, ml$ in hypoadrenocorticism. Diurnal variation in cortisol is lost in hyperadrenocorticism.
- Normally, Synacthen results in a rise in cortisol levels to over $18 \, \mu g/100 \, ml$. This rise is lost in hypoadrenocorticism (at an earlier stage in disease than the low cortisol level is found).
- Abdominal radiography may show calcified adrenals if tuberculosis is the cause of hypoadrenocorticism.
- Patients with Addison's disease may have various circulating autoantibodies.
- Plasma potassium is raised, sodium reduced in hypoadrenocorticism (converse in hyperadrenocorticism).

Other drugs

Particular note should be taken of anticoagulant and cardio-active drug use. Drug use may be an important pointer to underlying disease.

Drug abuse

This is discussed in Section 5.5.

3.5 Diabetes mellitus

Diabetes is a condition of impaired carbohydrate utilisation (impaired glucose tolerance) caused by insulin resistance or deficiency. This common condition affects some 4% of the population; only one half of these are diagnosed.

There are two main types of diabetics: juvenile onset and maturity onset (Table 3.10). The former presents a greater problem in management. Biochemical manifestations and commercial test reagents are listed in Table 3.11.

Table 3.10   Types of diabetes

	Type I (juvenile onset: insulin-dependent diabetes or IDD)	Type II (maturity onset: non insulin-dependent diabetes or NIDD)
Onset	Acute onset in childhood or adolescence	Slow onset in adult
Liability to ketosis	+ + +	+
Usual treatment	Diet + insulin	Diet ± oral hypoglycaemics

Table 3.11   Biochemical manifestations of diabetes

Manifestation	Comments	Commercial test reagents
Hyperglycaemia	Caused by impaired glucose metabolism	Dextrostix, BM stix, Glucostix
Glycosuria	Detectable when blood glucose increases to 10 mmol/litre as glucose spills over into urine	Clinistix, Diastix, Clinitest, Testape, BM test-5L
Ketosis	Fat is metabolised as energy source producing acetone, acetoacetate and β hydroxybutyrate (ketone bodies). Plasma bicarbonate is low	Ketostix
Ketonuria	Ketone bodies spill over into urine	Acetest

Clinical manifestations (see Section 4.7 for Emergencies)
- Cardiovascular: atherosclerosis.
- Ocular: retinopathy (cataracts).
- Renal: polyuria (renal failure).
- Neurological: peripheral and autonomic neuropathies.
- Others: infections; loss of consciousness.

Control of diabetes

- Diet should have a constant carbohydrate content, with the carbohydrate restricted at a level established as the diabetes is brought under control. Obese patients should have a reducing diet.
- Hypoglycaemic drugs are used mainly for maturity onset diabetics who cannot be controlled by diet alone. Glibenclamide or chlorpropamide are used for most NIDD under 65 years of age. Tolbutamide is used for older patients, and metformin for overweight patients.
- Insulin is given subcutaneously, often twice daily. Some patients can be controlled by a single daily injection of insulin zinc suspension lente (eg Humulin lente or Lentard), but if this is not possible using 52 units or more, a suitable alternative is a twice daily mixture of quick and intermediate acting insulins (Table 3.12). Exercise, surgery and infection increase insulin requirements.

The most certain but inconvenient way of assessing control is by serial measurements of blood glucose levels throughout the day. Usually, this is carried out by patients testing their urine at home and recording the degree of glycosuria with Clinitest tablets, Diastix or Diabus strips. Glycosuria tested in this relatively crude way does not usually became detectable until the blood sugar level is about 10 mmol/litre (which already represents a considerable degree of hyperglycaemia), and it is therefore important to

Table 3.12   Insulin preparations

Insulin preparation	Peak action (at h)	Duration of action (h)	Action
Humulins Actrapid Velosulin	2–4	6–10	Quick
Humulin I Insulated Monotard	4–10	18–24	Intermediate
Humulin lente Lentard	12–20	24–36	Long

assess the renal glucose threshold to ensure that the measurement of glycosuria is not misleading as to blood glucose levels. This can be roughly estimated by comparing simultaneous urine and blood sugar concentrations. The degree of ketosis can be rapidly assessed with Acetest tablets. A small amount of ketonuria, as shown by this test, is usually of no importance, but a strongly positive test, especially if confirmed by a positive ferric chloride reaction (Gerhardt's test), indicates a serious degree of ketosis. Confirmation is obtained by finding a low serum bicarbonate concentration. Glycosylated haemoglobin or fructosamine are usually monitored regularly to assess control. Non-diabetics have up to 7% glycosylated haemoglobin: 7–9% represents good control, over 13% shows poor control in diabetes.

Diagnosis

Diabetes is often detected at routine urinalysis by detecting glycosuria (±ketonuria). However, there are other causes of glycosuria (Table 1.16) and of ketonuria; diagnosis is therefore confirmed by blood glucose estimation (Table 3.13). Collect blood for this in the special fluoride-containing bottle (Table 1.21).

Diabetics do not always have glycosuria, so if this condition is suspected, always carry out blood glucose estimation. A random whole blood glucose over 10 mmol/litre or fasting level over about 6·7 mmol/litre usually establishes the diagnosis and glucose tolerance testing is seldom needed. (Plasma glucose levels are about 1 mmol/litre higher.)

Glucose tolerance testing is indicated only if blood sugar values are borderline.

Glucose tolerance test

A widely accepted simplified glucose tolerance test is as follows: give 75 g glucose orally, and take blood 2 hours later. A blood glucose level greater than 12 mmol/litre is diagnostic of diabetes; a blood glucose level of less than 7 mmol/litre excludes diabetes.

Table 3.13 Whole blood glucose estimation in diabetes

Diagnosis	Venous blood glucose levels (mmol/litre)	
	Fasting	Random
Non-diabetic	< 6	< 8
Diabetic	> 7	> 10

Management of diabetics undergoing dental surgery

The greatest danger to the patient is hypoglycaemia, because this produces neuroglycopenia. Under LA, always treat early in the morning. Always err on the side of hyperglycaemia.

Always consult the physician before considering general anaesthesia. Well controlled diabetics requiring a simple extraction under GA may be managed under a short outpatient GA early in the morning, if the patient is going to be able to eat normally soon afterwards. Admit the patient if in any doubt. Management of diabetics requiring a *long* operation under GA or of diabetics who are uncontrolled and require dental surgery under GA, must be discussed with the anaesthetist and the endocrine physician. Many regimes exist; two are outlined below. Always take blood 30 minutes preoperatively for laboratory assay of blood glucose levels, and arrange for diabetics to be tested early on in the operating list.

Regime A (Table 3.14)

Regime B – management of diabetics under GA

A method using an insulin pump together with a dextrose or saline IV infusion is popular in some centres, as it gives flexible control by varying the administration of insulin and/or dextrose (glucose).

A fast-acting insulin (eg Actrapid) is pumped, via an IV cannula, at about 4 units/hour. Simultaneously, 5% or 10% dextrose is infused at a rate that will produce a blood glucose level (monitored hourly by BM stix, or laboratory estimations) of about 8 mmol/litre.

3.6 Hyperparathyroidism

Hyperparathyroidism may cause
- Jaw radiolucencies/rarefaction.
- Loss of lamina dura.
- Giant cell granulomas (central).

The essential biochemical feature is a raised serum calcium level. This assay may need repeating several times to exclude hyperparathyroidism (Table 3.15). Blood for calcium levels should be collected:
- from fasting patient;
- early in the morning;
- with tourniquet off (venous stasis and fall in pH alter calcium levels);
- along with serum for albumin assay (albumin levels influence calcium levels).

Parathyroid hormone (PTH) levels should be assayed, but results may be

Table 3.14 Regime A[a] – management of diabetics under GA

	Non insulin-dependent[b]		Insulin-dependent (any operation)
	Minor operations, eg few extractions	Major operations, eg maxillofacial surgery	
Before operation	Stop biguanides. If on sulphonylurea, change to tolbutamide 7 days pre-op		Stabilise on at least twice daily insulin for 2–3 days pre-op. One day pre-op, use only short-acting insulin (Actrapid soluble or neutral)
During operation	Omit oral hypoglycaemic. Estimate blood glucose level	Do not give sulphonylurea or subcutaneous insulin on day of operation. Estimate blood glucose level. Set up intravenous infusion of 10% glucose 500 ml containing Actrapid or Leo neutral insulin 10 units plus KCl 1 g at 8.00 am. Infuse over 4 hours. Estimate blood glucose and potassium levels 2-hourly. Adjust insulin and potassium to keep blood glucose at 5–10 mmol/litre	
After operation	Estimate blood glucose up to 4 hours post-op	Continue infusion 4-hourly. Estimate blood glucose every 4 hours, potassium every 8 hours	
When resuming normal eating	Start sulphonylurea or other normal regimen	Stop infusion. Start Actrapid or Leo neutral insulin, and over the next 2 days:	
		Start sulphonylurea	Start normal insulin regimen

[a] Adapted, with permission, from Albertii and Thomas. *Br J Anaesth* 1979; **51:** 693.
[b] If well controlled; otherwise treat as insulin-dependent.

less helpful than calcium levels. PTH levels may be normal in some patients who have high calcium levels.

3.7 Genito-urinary and other infections (Tables 3.16; 3.17)

Sexually transmitted diseases

Imprecise diagnosis or empirical treatment serves only to spread these infections, as contact tracing is normally undertaken only on proven cases of sexually transmitted (venereal) disease. Failure to trace the contacts of an individual case not only swells the reservoir of infection, but may lead directly to disastrous clinical, family or social consequences to persons other than the patient. Treatment should never be instituted before

Table 3.15 Biochemical findings in disorders of calcium metabolism

Disease	Serum concentrations			
	Calcium	Phosphate	Alkaline phosphatase	Urea
Hyperparathyroidism				
Primary				
without osteitis fibrosa	↑[a]	↓	N	N
with osteitis fibrosa	↑	N or ↓	↑	N or ↑
Secondary				
due to renal failure	N or ↓	N or ↑	N or ↑	↑
due to malabsorption	N or ↓	↓	↑	N
Tertiary				
with osteitis fibrosa	↑	N or ↓	↑	N or ↑
without osteitis fibrosa	↑	↓	N	N or ↑
Hypoparathyroidism	↓	↑	N	N
Pseudohypoparathyroidism	↓	↑	N	N
Pseudopseudohypoparathyroidism	N	N	N	N
Vitamin D deficiency	↓	N or ↓	↑	N

[a] Arrows indicate values above↑ or below↓ normal (N).

Table 3.16 Infective diseases: incubation times and periods of infectivity

Disease	Incubation period	Period of infectivity[a]
Diphtheria	2–5 days	Until treated[b]
Gonorrhoea	2–5 days	Until treated
Scarlet fever	1–3 days	3 weeks after onset of rash
Measles	7–14 days	4 days after onset of rash
Pertussis	7–10 days	21 days after onset of symptoms
Chickenpox	14–21 days	Until all lesions scab
Mumps	12–21 days	7 days after onset of sialadenitis
Rubella	14–21 days	4 days after onset of rash
Hepatitis A	2–6 weeks	Usually non-infective at diagnosis
Hepatitis B	2–6 months	About 3 months after jaundice resolves[b]
Hepatitis non-A, non-B	?	?[b]
Human immunodeficiency virus	Up to at least 5 years	Persistent[b]
Infectious mononucleosis	30–50 days	?
Syphilis	9–90 days	Until treated

[a] Certain diseases are statutorily notifiable. Contact the microbiologist for further details.
[b] Carrier states exist.

bacteriological and/or serological specimens have been taken, and these specimens, or the results, should be referred with the patient to the nearest clinic for sexually transmitted diseases (Special Clinic or Genito-urinary Medicine Clinic).

Syphilis
- Dark field microscopy of a lesion may demonstrate *Treponema pallidum*. Wash oral lesions first with saline to remove oral commensal treponemes.
- Serology is indicated (Table 3.18). The VDRL is a screening test only, which may lead to false positives and therefore must be followed by a more specific test, such as the FTA-Abs or IgM-FTA-Abs.
- Always exclude other sexually transmitted diseases (STD), including hepatitis B.

Treatment.   Procaine penicillin for 10–21 days. In the penicillin-allergic patient, erythromycin or tetracycline.

Gonorrhoea
Gonococcal pharyngitis may be seen, particularly in homosexuals.
- Take a direct smear for Gram-staining (Gram-negative diplococci).
- Take a bacteriological swab from the area, for culture and sensitivities.
- Always also exclude syphilis and other STD.

Treatment.   Single dose of procaine penicillin with probenecid, or ampicillin with probenecid. In the penicillin-allergic patient, co-trimoxazole, cefuroxime or spectinomycin.

3.8 Acquired immune deficiency syndrome (AIDS) and other immunocompromised patients

AIDS is an uncommon disease of viral aetiology (Human Immunodeficiency Viruses HIV, of which there are at least HIV-1 and HIV-2). It affects predominantly male homosexuals, intravenous drug abusers, and, to a very much lesser extent, haemophiliacs, and consorts of HIV-positive patients.

AIDS is a severe immunodeficiency characterised by:
Opportunistic infections

Pneumonia, meningitis or encephalitis
  pneumocystis
  aspergillosis
  candidosis
  cryptococcosis

Table 3.17 Infectious diseases

Disease	Major manifestations	Oral manifestations	Laboratory diagnosis	Specific treatment used
AIDS (see Section 3.8)	Pneumonia, Kaposi's sarcoma	Candidosis, herpes simplex, hairy leukoplakia, periodontal disease, ulcers, Kaposi's sarcoma, cervical lymphadenopathy	Lymphopenia, HIV antibodies	None; zidovudine may prolong life
Cat scratch	Tender papule, regional lymph nodes enlarge, mild fever	Cervical lymphadenopathy	Leukocytosis, ESR raised. Skin test	None
Chickenpox (varicella)[a]	Rash evolves through macule, papule, vesicle and pustule; rash crops and is most dense on trunk	Oral ulcers	Complement fixation antibody titres (not usually needed)	Zoster immune globulin in high risk patients ±acyclovir
Cytomegalovirus[a]	Glandular fever type of syndrome (Paul-Bunnell negative)	—	Serology	None
Diphtheria	Tonsillar or pharyngeal exudate; cervical lymph nodes enlarged, myocarditis	Tonsillar exudate, palatal palsy	Culture Corynebacterium diphtheriae toxigenic strain	Antitoxin Penicillin
Erysipelas	Rash (confluent erythema and oedema)	—	Culture Streptococcus pyogenes	Penicillin
Hand, foot- and mouth disease	Rash, minor malaise	Oral ulceration (usually mild)	Serology	None
Hepatitis[a] (see Section 3.9)	Jaundice, malaise, pale stools, dark urine	—	Serology	Immune globulin in some patients
Herpangina	Fever, sore throat, enlarged cervical lymph nodes	Vesicles and ulcers on soft palate	Serology	None

Table 3.17 Infectious diseases—*contd*

Disease	Major manifestations	Oral manifestations	Laboratory diagnosis	Specific treatment used
Herpes simplex[a]	Fever, oral ulceration, gingivitis, cervical lymph node enlargement	Gingivostomatitis, herpes labialis (secondary infection)	Serology; viral isolation	Acyclovir
Herpes zoster[a] (shingles)	Rash like chickenpox but limited to dermatome, severe pain	Oral ulceration in zoster of maxillary or mandibular division of trigeminal nerve. Ulcers on palate and in pinna of ear in Ramsay-Hunt syndrome	Not needed	Acyclovir may help. Zoster immune globulin in high risk patients
Impetigo	Rash (bullous) spreading to other areas rapidly	Lesions on lips may resemble recurrent herpes labialis	Culture streptococci and/or staphylococci	Flucloxacillin
Infectious mononucleosis	Fever, lymph node enlargement, pharyngitis	Tonsillar exudate, palatal petechiae, oral ulceration	Blood film (atypical mononuclear cells), Monospot test, Paul-Bunnell test	None
Measles	Rash (maculopapular), fever, acute respiratory symptoms	Koplik's spots, pharyngitis	Not usually needed	Immune globulin in high risk patients
Mucocutaneous lymph node syndrome (Kawasaki disease)	Rash, hands and feet desquamation, lymph node enlargement, myocarditis	Strawberry tongue, labial oedema, pharyngitis	—	None
Mumps	Fever, malaise, parotitis	Sialadenitis, trismus, papillitis at salivary duct orifices	Complement fixing antibody titres to S and V antigens rise; not usually needed	None
Mycoplasmal pneumonia (atypical pneumonia)	Sore throat, fever, pneumonia	Erythema multiforme occasionally	Culture mycoplasma, complement fixing antibodies, cold agglutinins	Erythromycin or tetracycline

Table 3.17 Infectious diseases—*contd*

Disease	Major manifestations	Oral manifestations	Laboratory diagnosis	Specific treatment used
Pertussis[b] (whooping cough)	Cough, fever	Occasionally ulceration of lingual fraenum	Culture *Bordetella pertussis*	Ampicillin for secondary infection
Poliomyelitis	Paralyses	—	Serology	None
Rubella	Rash (mainly macular), fever, enlarged posterior cervical lymph nodes	Pharyngitis	Serology	None
Scarlet fever	Sore throat, fever, rash (macular), enlarged cervical lymph nodes, desquamation	Tonsillar punctate exudate, ± palatal petechiae, strawberry tongue	Culture *Streptococcus pyogenes* antistreptolysin O titre	Penicillin
Toxoplasmosis[a]	Glandular fever type of syndrome (Paul-Bunnell negative)	Sore throat	Sabin-Feldman dye test	Sulphonamide plus pyrimethamine

[a] Prevalent and often widespread infections in the immunocompromised high risk patients such as renal transplant or leukaemic patients.
[b] Some cases are caused by *Bordetella parapertussis*, or by viruses.

Table 3.18 Serological tests for syphilis

	Stage of disease					
	Primary		Secondary		Tertiary	
Test[a]	Untreated	Treated	Untreated	Treated	Untreated	Treated
Non-specific tests						
VDRL	Become +ve late	−ve	+ve	−ve	Usually +ve	+ve
Specific tests						
RPCFT,						
FTA-Abs,						
TPHA,						
TPI	Become +ve early	+ve	+ve	+ve	+ve	+ve

[a] See Appendix for explanation of abbreviations.

    nocardiosis
    zygomycosis (mucormycosis)
    strongyloidosis
    toxoplasmosis
    atypical mycobacteriosis
    cytomegalovirus
    herpes simplex

Brain
    progressive multifocal leukoencephalopathy
    polyoma JC virus

Chronic enterocolitis
    cryptosporidiosis
    isospra
    giardiasis

Malignant tumours

Mainly Kaposi's sarcoma.

Diagnosis is from clinical features, confirmed by finding lymphopenia and a severe T helper lymphocyte defect (actually, reduced OKT4+ or CD4+ cells) and HIV antibodies.
    Oral disease may include:

    Candidosis
    Herpetic infections

Hairy leukoplakia
Ulcers
Severe gingivitis or periodontitis
Kaposi's sarcoma
Lymphomas

Management is unsatisfactory; zidovudine (Retrovir) is the main drug used. Dental treatment may carry a risk of cross-infection and patients may have problems, including a bleeding tendency, and, of course, the patient is immunocompromised. Treatment should be carried out as for patients with hepatitis B (Section 3.9).

Note. Progressive generalised lymph node enlargement may be a manifestation of AIDS or a related syndrome.

If possible, avoid surgical extractions or any bone exposure. Minimise stripping of mucoperiosteum, and use chlorhexidine 0·2% mouthwash pre- and post-operatively. Consider antimicrobial prophylaxis.

Avoid paracetamol in those on zidovudine, since marrow suppression may be increased.

3.9 Hepatitis and liver disease

Liver disease is important in dental surgery because of (a) bleeding tendency, (b) drug intolerance, (c) possible viral hepatitis. The bleeding tendency may *sometimes* partly be reversed by vitamin K, 10 mg IM or IV daily.

Drug intolerance (Table 3.19) is a problem mainly in relation to general anaesthesia, but in patients with liver failure many drugs, even a small dose of diazepam, may be hazardous and can send the patient into a coma. Always consult the physician if you are considering dental treatment of an in-patient.

Viral hepatitis
Viral hepatitis B carries a small but significant mortality rate (1%) and a significant morbidity. Non-A, non-B hepatitis may also have similar morbidity and mortality (Table 3.20). The delta agent may be associated with hepatitis B, and carries a worse prognosis.

Hepatitis risk
Carrier states may complicate hepatitis B and non-A, non-B hepatitis. About 0·1% of the general population in North America, Northern Europe and the Antipodes are hepatitis B carriers.

Table 3.19   Drugs sometimes used in dentistry that may be contra-indicated in liver disease

Drug	Comment
Antidepressants	Avoid MAOI; reduce dose of others
Aspirin	Avoid; use paracetamol in reduced dose
Carbenoxolone	Avoid
Clindamycin	Avoid
Codeine	Avoid; use paracetamol in reduced dose
Erythromycin	Avoid the estolate ester
Etretinate	Avoid
Hypnotics	Avoid or use diazepam in reduced dose
Opiates	Avoid
Phenothiazines	Avoid
Sedatives	Avoid or use diazepam in reduced dose
Steroids	Avoid prednisone: use prednisolone
Suxamethonium	Avoid; may lead to prolonged apnoea
Tetracyclines	Avoid
Thiopentone	Avoid GA or use reduced dose

Note: General anaesthesia may be contra-indicated; repeated halothane administration may cause hepatitis.

Table 3.20   Comparative features of main types of viral hepatitis

	Hepatitis A (infectious hepatitis)	Hepatitis B (serum or Australian antigen hepatitis)	Non-A non-B hepatitis (hepatitis C)[a]
Incubation	2–6 weeks	2–6 months	2 weeks–2 months
Main route of transmission	Faecal–oral	Parenteral	Parenteral
Severity	Mild	May be severe	Moderate to severe
Complications	Rare	Small numbers chronic liver disease, hepatoma, polyarteritis nodosa, chronic glomerulonephritis	Small numbers chronic liver disease ? other
Carrier state possible	No	Yes	Yes
Mortality	0·1%	1–2%	?

[a] Several types.

Groups at high risk of hepatitis B carriage
- Patients with acute or chronic hepatitis.
- Normal patients who spent their childhood in countries outside Europe, North America, Australia and New Zealand, particularly those from Vietnam, etc.

- Drug addicts using injections, especially if suffering from hepatitis.
- Male homosexuals or bisexuals.
- Acute hepatitis in hospital staff.
- Acute hepatitis in inmates of mental institutions.
- Acute hepatitis more than 6 weeks after blood transfusion.
- Acute hepatitis in those who have been in countries outside Europe, North America, Australia or New Zealand between 6 weeks and 6 months previously.
- Chronic active hepatitis.
- Sexually promiscuous persons.

Screening patients for hepatitis B

If there is a high risk of the patient carrying hepatitis B virus, send a serum sample, taken with special precautions laid down for high-risk patients, as quickly as possible to the special laboratory for hepatitis B surface antigen screening. This test takes about 30 minutes. Until a report has been received, no further blood investigations should be carried out, unless these are very urgent and have been agreed with the pathologists concerned.

If the screening test is negative, it is probable that no further special precautions are necessary, unless there is some other infective risk, such as AIDS (Section 3.8) or non-A, non-B hepatitis. Screening does *not* totally exclude an infective risk: the presence of anti-HB$_c$ suggests infection.

Patients with positive tests for hepatitis B surface antigen (HB$_s$Ag) must be treated at this stage as high risk, and all blood samples must be taken with special precautions. The pathologist concerned should be consulted in advance, before any blood tests are requested, so that the range and frequency of laboratory investigations can be reduced to a minimum. The request form must be marked 'high risk'.

Patients positive for HB$_s$Ag should be screened for HB$_e$Ab (Table 3.21). About one in five are HB$_e$Ag positive. Those who have HB$_s$Ag should later be screened again at 3 months, and again if still positive. Those positive at 9 months are 'chronic carriers'.

Table 3.21   Interpretation of hepatitis B serology

Marker positive	Usual interpretation
HB$_s$Ag (surface antigen)	Virus present – infective risk
HB$_s$Ab (anti-HB$_s$Ag)	Immunity
HB$_e$Ag (e antigen)	High risk infectivity
HB$_e$Ab (anti-HB$_e$Ag)	No special high risk infection
HB$_a$Ab (anti-HB$_a$Ag)	Past or present infection

Dental treatment of a hepatitis B-positive or hepatitis-risk patient
Patients who are HB_eAb positive (and HB_eAg negative) are regarded as 'no special risk'; patients who are HB_eAb negative (but HB_eAg and HB_sAg positive) are a 'hepatitis risk' (Table 3.21).

Sterilisation of instruments

Use disposable equipment and materials wherever possible.
- Boiling water is inadequate.
- Autoclaving at 134°C for 3 minutes or hot air oven at 160°C for 1 hour are adequate.
- Effective disinfectants include:
  (1) Glutaraldehyde 2%. At least 30 minutes' exposure to fresh alkaline glutaraldehyde required. Solutions are toxic; take care not to carry glutaraldehyde over on to tissues.
  (2) Sodium hypochlorite 10%. At least 30 minutes' exposure required. Corrosive. Unstable in presence of cationic detergents.
  (3) Povidone-iodine (5000 ppm available iodine). At least 15 minutes' exposure required.

Control of cross-infection

All members of the dental team have a duty to ensure that all necessary steps are taken to prevent cross-infection, in order to protect their patients, colleagues and themselves. Provided adequate precautions are taken routinely, known carriers may be treated as a matter of course.

All tissues/body fluids are potentially infected. Most of the carriers of blood-borne viruses are not identified and they are unaware of their condition. It follows, therefore, that the routine practice adopted for *all* dental patients must be adequate enough to prevent cross-infection.

Apparently healthy carriers (including HIV-positive patients) should receive routine care. Immunocompromised patients need special care, to prevent them contracting infection as a result of receiving dental treatment.

Medical history – Identification of immunocompromised patients

- Individual chairside questioning should be used to identify any relevant medical history, including those likely to be immunocompromised.
- HBV and HIV screening of patients should *not* be undertaken as routine.
- Where the clinical condition of a patient warrants HBV (or HIV) testing, the information obtained will not alter the control of infection measures routinely adopted, except when a patient is immunocompromised.

- HIV testing, if indicated, should *first* be discussed with a senior member of staff, *before* suggesting the necessity to a patient. Referral to a specialist counsellor is required, prior to HIV testing.

Care of the immunocompromised

Immunocompromised groups to identify for special care:
- Those with known or suspected Acquired Immune Deficiency Syndrome (AIDS), or prodromal states;
- Those having immunosuppressive or cytotoxic therapy;
- Those on long-term corticosteroid therapy;
- Those with inherited disorders of immunity.

As these patients are extremely susceptible to infection, and may be at risk from the high counts of water-borne bacteria found in dental unit water systems, treatment must be carried out using dental units which have had their water systems decontaminated. This should be performed at the beginning of a treatment session, 1:1000 ppm chlorine solution being allowed to stand in the unit pipework for 10 minutes before flushing out with mains tap water.

Routine clinical practice – General comments

The routine measures introduced should be followed for every patient except the immunocompromised. The following recommendations are made in the light of current knowledge and may be subject to alteration and updating as further information becomes available.

A single tier system of patient management is introduced which will apply to all patients, and no patient's treatment should or need be delayed as a result of identification as a member of a 'risk group'.

All health-care workers are *strongly* advised to be immunised against hepatitis B if not already immune. They should also consider protection against other infectious diseases, such as diphtheria, poliomyelitis, tetanus, tuberculosis, and rubella (in the case of females).

No special measures are required by those who have not seroconverted after HBV immunisation, or who have not had HBV immunisation, as the routine measures when punctiliously carried out should afford all necessary protection. A patient should not be transferred to another person for treatment.

Clinical practice

Gloves should be worn routinely by all dentists, students, hygienists and close support dental staff. Wash hands before gloving, and after gloves are removed. Cuts and abrasions should be protected with waterproof dressings and/or double gloving as appropriate. Gloves must be changed if punctured and after treatment.

Masks and eye protection should be worn when aerosols or tooth fragments are generated. High volume aspiration must be used and waste should go into a central drain or sanitary suction unit. Care should be taken to ensure that the patient's eyes are adequately protected.

Clean white coats, or clean surgical gowns in surgical areas, must be worn. These must be changed if contaminated. Surgical gowns *must not* be taken into any food/drink area. Similarly, food/drink *must not* be consumed in clinical areas.

All 3-in-1 syringe tips, handpieces and ultrasonic scaler tips should be changed after use, and cleaned and autoclaved before re-use.

Ultrasound scaler handpiece ends, which cannot be sterilised, must be thoroughly cleaned and disinfected (eg with sanitiser solution) before re-use.

Cling-film should be placed across the dental chair control buttons operating light handles, ultrasonic scaler handpieces and 3-in-1 syringe bodies. The film must be changed or decontaminated with sanitiser solution after every patient.

Work surfaces in the operating area should be protected with cling-film or other disposable material and changed after every patient. The surface should then be sanitised.

Having positioned a patient ready for treatment, and fully equipped the operation area for the intended procedure, the operator should wash hands prior to gloving. From then, until the operative procedure is complete, the operator should avoid touching unprotected surfaces, the patient's notes, etc. Should extra instruments or other items be required, a non-operating assistant should perform these tasks.

All 'sharps' must *only* be disposed of in rigid-sided containers. This must include any steel burs, polishing cups or brushes, local anaesthetic cartridges, orthodontic wire, syringe needles, matrix bands and suture needles. The 'sharps' bins *must* be replaced when not more than two-thirds full.

Disposable polythene sleeving should be used routinely in oral surgery, for the pipes leading to the handpiece motor. This should be changed after every patient.

Benches and other work surfaces must not be used as seats.

Inoculation injuries are the most likely source of cross-infection. Re-sheathing of needles shall be avoided wherever possible. Where re-sheathing is necessary, this must be done using one hand only; resheathing devices designed to protect against inoculation injury should be used.

When cleaning an operation area or instruments, heavy-duty gloves should be worn.

All grinding stones, diamond burs, etc, should be cleaned (wearing gloves) and sterilised by autoclaving.

Laboratory procedures

The principle involved is that impressions and other items received by a laboratory should have been decontaminated in the clinical area concerned. All items should leave a laboratory clean and decontaminated.

Clinical procedures

Before despatch to a laboratory, *all* impressions and other items which have intra-oral contamination should be thoroughly rinsed in running tap water and then spray disinfected with 0·5% aqueous chlorhexidine solution. Items should not be covered with napkins, but should be placed in a polythene bag, so that the items can be inspected externally.

Items received from a laboratory must be thoroughly washed in running tap water before further handling.

Laboratory reception

Laboratories should establish a receiving area separate from the production and despatch areas. Laboratory coats and gloves should be worn. Items should be inspected through the unopened polythene bag when they are received. Obvious blood contamination requires that the unopened item be returned to the clinical area concerned for correct decontamination and re-bagging.

Satisfactory items should be removed from the bag and thoroughly washed in running tap water before handling. Dispose of the polythene bag in yellow, bag-lined waste bins.

Decontaminate work surfaces in the reception area daily (wearing gloves); use disposable towelling and sanitiser solution.

Production areas

Use safety equipment or wear safety glasses and masks whilst working, as appropriate. Keep work surfaces clean and use clean instruments, attachments and materials for the construction of items manufactured in the laboratory.

Change pumice daily and form a slurry with alcoholic chlorhexidine solution (0·2%). Clean and disinfect brushes, wheels and mops daily.

Items which have been in a patient's mouth should be handled separately from new, uncontaminated items. Separate sets of instruments, wheels, brushes, pumice troughs, etc, should be dedicated to each type of case, wherever possible.

Despatch area
Partly constructed items should be thoroughly washed and bagged, ready for despatch to a clinical area.

Finished items should be washed, decontaminated with 0·5% aqueous chlorhexidine spray and sealed in a polythene bag, ready for despatch to a clinic. Attach a warning label to remind the clinician to wash the item before insertion into a patient's mouth.

In the event of accidental injury to operator
(1) Ensure that the accident is not repeated.
(2) Wash the wound.
(3) Test the patient's serum for hepatitis B antigens and enquire about possible HIV positivity.
(4) If the patient's serum is negative, there is probably no problem.
(5) If the patient's serum is positive for hepatitis B, consult a microbiologist for advice concerning hepatitis B immunoglobulin and/or vaccination against hepatitis B. If HIV is involved, consult a microbiologist.

Hepatitis B vaccine
Hepatitis B vaccine consists of HB_sAg. Vaccination gives apparently protective antibody levels after three doses in 85–95% of healthy adults. The antibody persists for at least 3 years; boosters may be needed later, probably by 5 years. Most of those who have not received protection after vaccination have been patients who were already in the incubation phase of hepatitis B, were over 50 years of age, were on renal haemodialysis, were obese, or were immunocompromised.

Vaccination is not needed in those who are HB_sAb positive (but is not harmful to such individuals). It is ineffective in chronic HB_sAg carriers. There are no known serious immediate or long-term complications, and pregnancy is not a contra-indication to vaccination in a mother at high risk of hepatitis B, since the risks to mother and foetus from hepatitis B infection are serious.

Hepatitis B vaccine is currently recommended for persons at high risk:
- Male homosexuals and bisexuals.
- Abusers of intravenous drugs.
- Institutionalised mentally handicapped patients.
- Refugees from areas with high endemic disease (eg, the Third World, and especially Vietnam).

- Haemodialysis patients.
- Recipients of blood clotting factor concentrates.
- Close contacts of HB$_s$Ag carriers.
- Selected health care workers, including clinical dental staff.

3.10 Pregnancy

Points to remember:
- Pregnancy is the ideal opportunity to begin preventive dental education.
- Drugs and radiation should be avoided whenever possible during pregnancy (see Section 1.3 and Table 3.22), particularly the first trimester.

Table 3.22   Drugs used in dentistry which may be contra-indicated in pregnancy

Drugs to avoid	First trimester	Second and third trimesters	Close to delivery	During lactation[a]
Aminoglycosides		+		
Anticoagulants[b]	+		+	+
Antifibrinolytics	+	+	+	
Aspirin			+	+
Atropine				+
Barbiturates		+		
Benzodiazepines[c]		+	+	+
Chloral hydrate				+
Corticosteroids[d]		+	+	+
Co-trimoxazole			+	
Danazol	+	+	+	+
Diflunisal				+
Erythromycin				+
Etretinate	+	+	+	
Gentamicin		+		
Mefenamic acid		+	+	
Metronidazole	+			+
Opiates[e]			+	
Penicillin				+
Phenothiazines				+
Rifampicin			+	
Sulphonamides		+	+	+
Tetracyclines		+	+	+
Tricyclics		+	+	

+ = Avoid especially at these times.
[a] These and other drugs enter the breast milk and could in theory harm the infant.
[b] Oral anticoagulants.
[c] If these are necessary, use a short-acting drug, eg temazepam.
[d] Systemic corticosteroids.
[e] Including related compounds, eg codeine, dihydrocodeine, pentazocine and pethidine.

- In general, most treatment is best carried out in the 4th to 6th month of pregnancy (second trimester).
- In the third trimester, avoid GA because of the liability of vomiting and do not lay the patient supine, as this may cause hypotension.

3.11 Patients with malignant disease, including those on radiotherapy or chemotherapy

Discussing the disease

It is always a problem to know how much to tell a patient who has cancer. If a patient asks a direct question, using the word cancer or a more technical synonym, one must presume that they have considered the implications and expect a truthful answer. It is usually wise to explain that there are many kinds of tumour, some of which can be completely eradicated and others quite effectively treated, but it is wise to refer questions to senior colleagues.

Few patients do actually ask the direct question, and it is usually wrong to volunteer too much pathological information; however, do ask them whether there is anything that they would like to ask.

In many instances, investigations are carried out on patients to exclude the presence of a cancer, and if cancer is excluded from the differential diagnosis, it is part of good management to tell patients and their relatives that they need no longer worry about cancer. At least one of the responsible relatives should always be told the complete truth. Compassion will lead most families to request that the patient is kept in ignorance, and most patients who know their diagnosis will ask that their families are spared the full truth.

Effects of treatment on the oral tissues

Surgical treatment of malignant neoplasms in the head and neck is inevitably disfiguring to some degree, but cosmetic results are continually being improved and much can be offered. Rapidly proliferating epithelium such as the oral mucosa is highly susceptible to the cytotoxic action of chemotherapeutic drugs and radiation used in the treatment, with epithelial thinning, erythema, sloughing and a susceptibility to ulceration and infection. Mucosal damage is usually self-limiting, and heals in two to three weeks without scarring.

Direct effects on mucosa are swift to follow the administration of:

- methotrexate
- 5-fluorouracil

- bleomycin
- cytosine arabinoside
- doxorubicin (adriamycin)

The salivary glands are directly affected by radiation, resulting in saliva of:

- decreased volume
- lower pH
- increased viscosity
- altered composition

Salivary gland injury is slow in onset, but correspondingly longer in recovery, with a possibility of permanent damage. Many patients adopt a soft carbohydrate diet, which leads to a greatly increased caries rate. Cervical margin and cuspal caries are common.

During chemotherapy the oral flora changes to faecal types, and the overall swing is to Gram-negative organisms. There might be infection with fungi, and the decreased immune competence of the patient makes viral infection likely (notably herpes types).

Indirect effects of cytotoxics on the bone marrow may result in:

- Leukopenia and neutropenia – infection.
- Thrombocytopenia – haemorrhage/bleeding tendency.
- A platelet count of less than 20×10^9/litre will probably give rise to ecchymoses of the floor of the mouth and spontaneous gingival bleeding.
- Anaemia.
- Endarteritis obliterans – risk of osteoradionecrosis.
- Neurotoxicity – pain.
- Pain in the mandibular teeth without pulpal involvement is a (rare) complication of vincristine use.

Other adverse effects of cytotoxic agents may include:

- nausea and vomiting;
- diarrhoea;
- alopecia;
- infertility;
- depression;
- pulmonary fibrosis and Raynaud's syndrome with bleomycin;
- impaired renal function, especially with cisplatin;
- cystitis with ifosfamide and cyclophosphamide;
- damage to the VIII cranial nerve with cisplatin;
- cardiotoxicity with doxorubicin and daunorubicin especially.

Management

The newly diagnosed patient who has just been told that he/she has cancer will be in a state of mental turmoil and not able to assimilate much of what is said. It is quite likely that he/she will fail to see the importance of the oral examination. There is no point in unkind criticism of the patient who has poor oral hygiene, but it is absolutely essential that he/she understands the risks and discomfort which will ensue if meticulous oral hygiene is not maintained.

Some malignant diseases, such as childhood leukaemias and adult Hodgkin's, can now be cured, so the most important consideration with regard to dental treatment is whether the patient is about to have, or has undergone, a course of treatment which is intended to be curative ('radical') or palliative.

Discuss the prognosis with the responsible oncologist or radiotherapist. Heroic removal of teeth and bridge-planning is obviously inappropriate for a patient who has a poor life expectancy, but that does not mean that quality of life can be ignored. Elimination of pain and infection, and even provision of dentures, can make a great difference to the patient's psychological state.

Interest and care should be the aim of all staff involved.

General assessment
- A full history and examination of the head, neck, mouth and perioral tissues (Table 3.23).
- Radiographs: panoramic and bitewings or oblique lateral mandibles and bitewings, plus intra-orals to augment the above.

Table 3.23   TNM classification of malignant neoplasms[a]

Primary tumour (T)	
T_0	No evidence of primary tumour
T_{is}	Carcinoma *in situ*
T_1, T_2, T_3	Increasing size of tumour[b]
Regional lymph nodes (N)	
N_0	Regional lymph node not clinically demonstrable
N_{1a}, N_{2a}	Demonstrable regional nodes; a = no metastases 1 = unilateral movable; 2 = contralateral or bilateral movable
N_{1b}, N_{2b}	Demonstrable regional nodes; b = metastases suspected
N_3	Fixed nodes
N_x	Regional nodes cannot be assessed clinically
Distant metastases (M)	
M_0	No evidence of distant metastases
M_1, M_2, M_3	Increasing degrees of metastatic involvement, including distant nodes

[a]Several other classifications are available, eg STNM (S = site).
[b]T_1 maximum diameter 2 cm; T_2 maximum diameter of 4 cm; T_3 maximum diameter over 4 cm.

- Full blood and platelet count, haemostatic screening tests and liver function tests. There may be anaemia and/or bleeding tendency.

Oral hygiene

Gentle, constant reiteration of oral hygiene with instruction and supervision by a dental hygienist, and scaling and polishing, will be not only valuable but will be appreciated as part of the general care. The patient should be provided with 0·2% aqueous chlorhexidine mouthrinses.

Pain

Potential sources of pain, eg carious teeth, should be treated or extracted, as appropriate. Pain from ulceration can be relieved by hot saline mouthwashes, lignocaine or benzydamine 0·15% (Difflam Oral Rinse) 10 ml mouthrinse 1-hourly, reducing to 2- to 3-hourly as the pain abates.

Deep pain needs systemic analgesia; do not hesitate to prescribe narcotics such as morphine sulphate to patients with terminal malignancy.

Refer patients to a pain relief clinic or hospice as required.

Management before surgery for oral cancer
(1) Assess tumour invasion, especially bone and nodes.
(2) Plan care of dentition (see below).
(3) Group and cross-match 4 units of blood.
(4) ECG is usually indicated as well as the above investigations.
(5) Book intensive care unit.
(6) Informed consent extends to warning the patient that he/she will have procedures such as tracheotomy and will awaken in ITU.

Management before cytotoxic chemotherapy or radiotherapy
- Meticulous oral hygiene; professional cleaning (if platelet counts are high enough to permit).
- Elimination of causes of irritation:
  (*a*) remove appliances, including orthodontic bands and retainers;
  (*b*) smooth sharp teeth or fillings (or extract tooth).
- Elimination of potential sources of infection:
  (*a*) remove overhanging crowns or filling margins;
  (*b*) extract doubtful teeth;
  (*c*) extract teeth with deep periodontal pockets;
  (*d*) extract partially erupted third molars (excise operculum as a temporary measure).
- Corticosteroid mouthwashes may reduce radiation mucositis (see Table 3.24)

Table 3.24 Oral complications of radiotherapy

Complication	Management
Mucositis	Prophylaxis; Betnesol 0·5 mg tablets as a mouthwash four times daily from the day before radiotherapy, throughout the course Warm normal saline mouth baths *or* 0·2% aqueous chlorhexidine mouth baths
Ulcers	0·2% aqueous chlorhexidine mouth baths four times daily
Candidosis	Nystatin suspension 100 000 u/ml as mouth wash four times daily
Xerostomia	Saliva substitute[a] Frequent sips of water
Caries	Daily topical fluoride applications (see Section 9.2) Avoid sugary diet
Dental hypersensitivity	Fluoride applications
Periodontal disease	Oral hygiene 0·2% aqueous chlorhexidine mouth baths
Loss of taste	—
Trismus	Jaw-opening exercises three times daily
Osteoradionecrosis/ irradiation-induced osteomyelitis	Avoid by planned pre-radiotherapy extractions or extractions within 3 months of radiotherapy, and atraumatic extractions under antibiotic cover

[a]Artificial saliva, eg methyl cellulose, hypromellose or polyethylene oxide (300 mg Polyox tablets sucked with a little water).

Surgery

Tooth extraction, or other surgical procedures should be done *before* chemotherapy is started, because of the risk of serious infection when the bone marrow is suppressed. There is less urgency if radiotherapy is planned and, in the case of third molars, it might be better to wait for the end of the course before their removal. Modern radiotherapy methods give rise to less obliterative endarteritis than formerly, but it is unwise to delay surgery for longer than 6 months after radiotherapy.

Management of patients on cytotoxics or having radiotherapy

Infections are potentially life-threatening in the immunosuppressed patient, and most antibiotic regimes suitable for ordinary dental bacterial infections are inadequate. A very broad-spectrum cover is needed (such as penicillin plus gentamicin). Swab culture is often unsatisfactory, since a wide range of organisms can contribute to the infection. Ask the advice of a microbiologist. Acyclovir 5 mg/kg by slow IV infusion over 1 hour, repeated 8-hourly, is indicated for severe herpes virus infections; topical and oral preparations are now available (Section 5.7). Fungal infections are discussed in Section 5.7.

Haemorrhage, whether spontaneous or post-operative, needs the advice of a haematologist. If it is due to thrombocytopenia, a platelet transfusion might be indicated, plus tranexamic acid 1 g 2–4 times daily. A tranexamic acid mouthwash may help.

Radiotherapy involving the oral tissues may give rise to a range of complications, whereas the main problem with cytotoxic chemotherapy is oral ulceration (Table 3.24; see also Table 3.4).

Avoid aspirin and other NSAIDS in patients on methotrexate as toxicity of the latter is increased.

Cytotoxic agents and regimens

Some of the miscellany of agents and regimens are outlined in Tables 3.25 and 3.26.

3.12 Renal disease

Renal patients may have impaired drug excretion, a problem mainly when general anaesthesia is contemplated. Consult the physician (see also Tables 3.27 and 5.22–5.24). Avoid NSAIDS and tetracyclines.

The other main problems are in relation to the immunosuppression created following a kidney transplant and a bleeding tendency. Organise dental treatment *before* the transplant.

3.13 Respiratory disease

Points to remember:
- Respiratory disease is common.
- Upper respiratory tract infections (eg common cold) are a contra-indication to non-urgent general anaesthesia, because the infection may be spread to the lower respiratory tract. Lower respiratory tract infections are a contra-indication to GA.
- General anaesthesia is potentially hazardous in patients with respiratory disease, because respiratory failure may be precipitated. Post-operative pulmonary complications are also more likely in this group.
- If possible, avoid general anaesthesia and respiratory depression. Reduce or avoid sedatives and analgesics.

3.14 Transplants and prostheses

Transplants

Transplants of many kinds are commonplace today, especially renal transplants. Patients with transplants are, particularly during the immediate post-operative period, liable to present a number of complications to dental treatment; in particular:

- need for a corticosteroid cover;
- liability to infection;
- bleeding tendency (if on anticoagulants);
- gingival hyperplasia if on cyclosporin.

Dental treatment should be carried out in close consultation with the physicians/surgeons responsible for the patient and, in many instances, would be better performed pre-operatively.

Oral health is important in these patients, who are particularly liable to the same fungal and viral infections and other complications seen in patients on chemotherapy for malignant disease (see Section 3.11).

Bone marrow transplants may produce graft versus host disease, manifesting with lichen planus or Sjögren's syndrome.

Erythromycin is contra-indicated since it decreases cyclosporin metabolism and increases its toxicity.

Prostheses

Prostheses are also commonplace, particularly cardiac valvular prostheses, prosthetic joints, and ventriculo-atrial shunts (for hydrocephalus).

Cardiac prostheses and pacemakers

Patients with cardiac prostheses and those with pacemakers clearly have underlying cardiac disorders, which may be a contra-indication to general anaesthesia. Patients with prostheses have additional problems in relation to bleeding tendency (anticoagulants: Section 3.2, and infective endocarditis: Section 3.3).

Patients with pacemakers may be in danger in relation to the use of equipment which may interfere with their pacemaker, such as diathermy, electrosurgery, ultrasonic scalers, and pulp testers.

Prosthetic joints

There is no good evidence for infection of these prostheses arising from oral sepsis. However, since there is perhaps a theoretical risk that the bacteraemia associated with tooth extraction might lead to metastatic infection, it seems reasonable to give an antimicrobial cover if the orthopaedic surgeon wishes (see Section 5.7).

Table 3.25   Cytotoxic regimens

	MOPP	MVPP	ChlVPP	ABVD	CVB	CHOP
	Hodgkin's lymphoma	Hodgkin's lymphoma	Hodgkin's lymphoma	Hodgkin's lymphoma	Hodgkin's lymphoma	Non-Hodgkin's lymphoma
Nitrogen mustard	+	+	−	−	−	−
Vincristine	+	−	−	−	−	+
Procarbazine	+	+	+	−	−	−
Prednisone	+	+	+	−	−	+
Vinblastine	−	+	+	+	+	−
Chlorambucil	−	−	+	−	−	−
Adriamycin	−	−	−	+	−	+
Bleomycin	−	−	−	+	+	−
DTIC	−	−	−	+	−	−
CCNU	−	−	−	−	+	−
Cyclophosphamide	−	−	−	−	−	+
Cytarabine	−	−	−	−	−	−
Methotrexate	−	−	−	−	−	−
5-Fluorouracil	−	−	−	−	−	−
Cisplatin	−	−	−	−	−	−
Actinomycin D	−	−	−	−	−	−

Table 3.25   Cytotoxic regimens—*contd*

	COAP	CMF	VAC (DOC)	VAC-A	PVB	VAB
	Acute myeloid leukaemia	Breast carcinoma	Ewing's sarcoma	Ewing's sarcoma	Testicular carcinoma	Testicular carcinoma
Nitrogen mustard	−	−	−	−	−	−
Vincristine	+	−	+	+	−	−
Procarbazine	−	−	−	−	−	−
Prednisone	+	−	−	−	−	−
Vinblastine	−	−	−	−	+	+
Chlorambucil	−	−	−	−	−	−
Adriamycin	−	−	+	+	−	−
Bleomycin	−	−	−	−	+	+
DTIC	−	−	−	−	−	−
CCNU	−	−	−	−	−	−
Cyclophosphamide	+	+	+	+	−	+
Cytarabine	+	−	−	−	−	−
Methotrexate	−	+	−	−	−	−
5-Fluorouracil	−	+	−	−	−	−
Cisplatin	−	−	−	−	+	+
Actinomycin D	−	−	−	−	−	+

Table 3.26   Other cytotoxic agents

Agent	Used in	Agent	Used in
Amsacrine	Acute leukaemias, lymphomas	Lomustine	Lymphoma
Busulphan	Chronic myeloid leukaemia	Melphalan	Myeloma
Carboplatin	Germ cell neoplasms	Mercaptopurine	Acute leukaemia
Carmustine	Lymphoma	Mitobronitol	Chronic myeloid leukaemia
Dacarbazine	Melanoma	Mitomycin	Lymphoma
Doxorubicin (adriamycin)	Various neoplasms	Mitozantrone	Breast carcinoma
Epirubicin	Various neoplasms	Mustine	Lymphoma
Estramustine	Prostatic carcinoma	Razoxane	Sarcoma
Ethoglucide	Bladder carcinoma	Thioguanine	Acute leukaemia
Etoposide	Choriocarcinoma	Thiotepa	Meningeal cancer
Hydroxyurea	Chronic myeloid leukaemia	Treosulfan	Ovarian carcinoma
Ifosfamide	Lymphoma	Vindesine	Acute leukaemia

Ventriculo-atrial shunts

The complications of infection of these valves (eg Spitz–Holter valve) are so serious that, although as in the case of prosthetic joints there is little evidence for an oral source, it seems reasonable to give an antimicrobial cover, after consultation with the responsible neurosurgeon.

3.15 Other relevant conditions

Every condition which is elicited from the medical history should be checked for relevance in a standard text, but the following can be highly relevant (see also Tables 5.22–5.24):

- *Malignant hyperthermia* (malignant hyperpyrexia): various general anaesthetics and other agents may be contra-indicated.
- *Porphyria*: intravenous barbiturates, metronidazole and other agents may be contra-indicated.
- *Suxamethonium sensitivity*: suxamethonium is contra-indicated.
- *Hereditary angioedema*: any dental trauma may result in oedema and a hazard to the airway. Stanozolol may be indicated pre-operatively.
- *Rheumatoid arthritis*: cervical spine involvement may predispose to spinal cord damage if the neck is flexed during general anaesthesia.

Table 3.27 Drugs used in dentistry which may be contra-indicated in patients with chronic renal failure[a]

Safe		Reduce dose		Dangerous
No dosage change usually required	Only in severe renal failure	Dosage reduction indicated[b] except in mild renal failure	Even in mild renal failure	Best avoided in any patient with renal failure
Clindamycin	Ampicillin	Cephalosporins[c]	Acyclovir[d]	Aspirin
Cloxacillin	Amoxycillin	Pancuronium	Gentamicin	Cephaloridine
Diazepam	Barbiturates	Paracetamol	Streptomycin	Cephalothin
Doxycycline	Benzylpenicillin	Tubocurarine	Vancomycin	Diflunisal
Erythromycin	Co-trimoxazole			NSAIDS
Minocycline	Codeine			Sulphadiazine
	Lincomycin			Tetracyclines[e]
	Metronidazole			
	Opiates			
	Phenothiazines			
	Sulphonamides			

Note: General anaesthesia may be contra-indicated.

[a] Many other drugs unlikely to be used in dentistry may be contra-indicated: check the literature.

[b] Severe renal failure – GFR < 10 ml/minute; moderately severe renal failure – GFR < 25 ml/minute; mild renal failure – GFR < 50 ml/minute.

[c] Except cephaloridine and cephalothin which are contra-indicated.

[d] Systemic acyclovir.

[e] Except doxycycline and minocycline.

● Athletes: the International Olympic Committee (IOC) prohibits the use of various drugs by athletes. Antimicrobials are allowed, and analgesics such as aspirin and paracetamol are permitted alone, but codeine and dextropropoxyphene are banned. Anxiolytics may sometimes be banned, and ephedrine and systemic corticosteroids are best avoided. Topical corticosteroids are permitted.

4

Emergencies

Emergencies should be prevented where possible, but, in any event, staff should be trained in their management and a kit readily available. This should contain:

- Apparatus for giving oxygen;
- Oral airway;
- Tourniquet, syringes and needles;
- Aspirator;
- Sugar such as glucose solution for oral use;
- Drugs for injection;
  - (a) 50% sterile glucose;
  - (b) 1 in 1000 adrenaline;
  - (c) 100–200 mg hydrocortisone succinate;
  - (d) 10 mg diazepam

4.1 Respiratory obstruction

Complete respiratory obstruction rapidly leads to cerebral hypoxia and, after about three minutes, to brain damage and death. Its management is discussed in Chapter 8.

Respiratory obstruction in relation to dental surgery occurs mainly in the following ways.

Mechanical obstruction by an object in the airway

It is a relatively common error to collect extracted teeth in a swab and then by mistake use that swab again post-operatively, transferring removed teeth back into the mouth. Unfortunately, it is also only too common that inlays, crowns and endodontic instruments continue to be dropped into the airway; use of rubber dam reduces these mishaps.

Management of an inhaled foreign body

If the patient cannot cough the object out, he should not be slapped on the back. This might actually permit an object to fall further into the respiratory tract. The Heimlich manoeuvre may clear the airway (fig. 4.1) but, failing this, the object must be removed by endoscopy.

Pressure on the airway
This may be due to laryngeal oedema (trauma, infection or acute angiooedema), impacted middle third facial fracture, or the tongue falling into the pharynx, bleeding into fascial spaces of the neck, or a tumour.

Management of pressure on the airway
If the cause cannot be treated tracheotomy may become necessary (see Chapter 8).

Acute asthmatic attack

Management of acute asthmatic attack
The patient should use his normal bronchodilator (usually salbutamol, fenoterol or ipratropium bromide), but it may be necessary to give oxygen, steroids (hydrocortisone 200 mg IV immediately) and a sympathomimetic

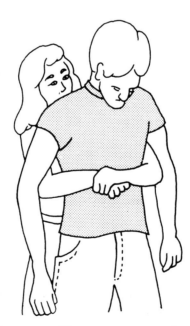

Fig. 4.1 The Heimlich manoeuvre. The operator grasps one fist with the opposite hand and rapidly presses inwards and upwards.

agent (either salbutamol 2·5 mg or terbutaline 5 mg by nebuliser) (see Section 4.10). Aminophylline 250 mg given slowly IV over 15 minutes is an alternative sympathomimetic bronchodilator and is preferable to adrenaline, but in any event call a physician immediately to deal with this.

4.2 Material lost from the mouth

If material such as an extracted tooth cannot be found lying free in the mouth, it can either be outside the body or within the body, in the oral tissues, gastrointestinal tract, or respiratory tract. The following procedures are advisable:
(1) Check carefully every accessible site.
(2) If the object cannot be found, take a plain abdominal radiograph and chest radiographs (two views at right angles).
(3) Direct bronchoscopy may well be more successful than chest radiography in locating an inhaled foreign body.

4.3 Emergencies in dentistry

Emergencies in dentistry are summarised in Table 4.1.

4.4 Collapse

Causes of collapse include syncope, myocardial infarction/cardiac arrest, bradycardia or heart block, hypoglycaemia, stroke, corticosteroid insufficiency, epilepsy, anaphylaxis, drug reaction, and hysteria.

Syncope

Syncope is loss of consciousness caused by cerebral ischaemia. Causes include:
- faint (vasovagal attack);
- postural hypotension;
- severe haemorrhage;
- acute cardiac failure; cardiac arrest, heart block (Stokes-Adams attacks).

Fainting

Where possible, avoid faints by:
- Ensuring the patient eats before treatment under local analgesia.
- Adopting a reassuring manner and not causing undue anxiety.
- Laying the patient supine *before* any injections.
- Not causing the patient pain.

Table 4.1 Summaries of management of collapse in dentistry

Cause	Clinical features	Precipitating factors	Management
Faint	Dizziness, weakness, nausea, pallor, cold moist skin (clammy), pulse initially slow and weak	Anxiety, pain, fatigue, fasting, high temperature	Lower patient's head (lay him flat). Recovery is usually rapid – within seconds (± smelling salts)
Hypoglycaemia	Drowsiness, disorientation, irritability, aggression, warm moist skin, pulse full and rapid	Lack of food, too much insulin	Lay patient flat Give glucose orally (4 sugar or dextrose lumps or glucose drink) or intravenously (50 ml 50% sterile glucose) Get medical assistance
Cardiac arrest	Loss of consciousness, cessation of respiration, absence of arterial pulses, pallor or cyanosis	Myocardial infarction, hypoxia, anaesthetic overdose	Summon medical assistance Lay patient flat on hard surface Give blow to sternum Start cardiopulmonary resuscitation
Stroke	Loss of consciousness, hemiplegia	Hypertension	Maintain airway
Corticosteroid insufficiency	Loss of consciousness, pulse weak and rapid, falling blood pressure	Stress of trauma in patient on steroids	Lay patient flat Give methylprednisolone 500 mg or hydrocortisone 500 mg intravenously Give oxygen Summon medical assistance

Table 4.1 Summaries of management of collapse in dentistry—*contd*

Cause	Clinical features	Precipitating factors	Management
Epilepsy	Loss of consciousness, widespread jerking, sometimes incontinence	Some drugs, starvation, menstruation	Lay patients in head injury position Stop them damaging themselves. Maintain airway If not recovered in 5 minutes, give diazepam 0·1 mg/kg IV or midazolam 2 mg IV every minute.
Anaphylaxis	Loss of consciousness, cold clammy skin, pulse weak and rapid, oedema/urticaria/wheeze, falling blood pressure	Exposure to allergen, eg penicillin	Lay patient flat Give 1 ml 1:1000 adrenaline intramuscularly. Give hydrocortisone sodium succinate 200–500 mg IM or IV or methylprednisolone 500 mg IV. Give oxygen Summon medical assistance
Suspected drug reaction	Variably confusion, drowsiness, fits or loss of consciousness	Drugs	Lay patient flat Maintain airway Summon medical assistance
Hysteria	Often a female patient. Variable hyperventilation, crying, etc.	Anxiety	Exclude organic reactions (above) Reassure

Unless laid flat, a fainting patient may develop cerebral hypoxia and then convulse. If he or she does not immediately recover on being laid flat, check the pulse. If slow, this may suggest a vasovagal attack, which might respond to atropine (Table 4.1). If the pulse is absent, this represents cardiac arrest (see Section 4.6).

Management of collapse (Table 4.1)

Postural hypotension
Rapidly bringing a patient upright from lying down may produce postural hypotension, particularly under the following conditions:
- After prolonged periods lying down.
- In the elderly.
- In those on anti-hypertensive drugs, tricyclic antidepressants or other drugs with an atropinic action.

Paradoxically, the converse may occur late in pregnancy, if the gravid uterus inhibits venous return to the heart when the patient lies down (supine hypotensive syndrome).

4.5 Bleeding

Life-threatening acute haemorrhage from oral or perioral vessels is very uncommon, but severe haemorrhage may follow damage to vessels such as the maxillary artery (see also Chapter 8). Patients who have had radical neck dissections (eg those with malignancy) may occasionally have acute life-threatening haemorrhage from erosion of the carotid artery under an infected flap.

Manifestations of bleeding include falling blood pressure (BP), rising pulse rate and collapse. Investigations include:
- Haemoglobin. Shortly after haemorrhage no abnormality is found but, as over a few hours haemodilution occurs, the haemoglobin level falls.
- Haematocrit (packed cell volume, PCV) also falls.
- Central venous pressure (CVP) is more sensitive to blood volume loss than is the BP (Chapter 7).
- Urine output is reduced (and if the BP remains low, acute renal failure may supervene).

Management
- Prevent further blood loss by direct pressure.
- Take blood for haemoglobin levels, grouping and cross-matching.
- Set up an IV infusion (Section 7.9).
- Transfuse to restore blood volume if indicated (Section 7.10). ·

4.6 Cardiac arrest

Recognition
- Sudden loss of consciousness.
- Absent arterial pulses (carotid or femoral).
- Gasping or absent respiration (after 15–30 seconds) – a *late* sign.
- Pupils begin to dilate after about 90 seconds.

Immediate treatment
- Call for assistance.
- Sharp blow to pericardium; may restart heart in asystole.
- Clear and maintain airway; inflate with oxygen.
- Institute cardiopulmonary resuscitation (Table 4.2) (external cardiac compression plus artificial ventilation).
- Give intravenous infusion of 8·4% sodium bicarbonate, giving 100 ml (100 mmol) over 10 to 15 minutes to combat acidosis.

4.7 Diabetes (see also Section 3.5)

Collapse
Collapse in a diabetic may be caused by:
- abnormal blood sugar (glucose) levels (hypoglycaemia or hyperglycaemia);
- other causes, eg faint or cardiac arrest.

Hypoglycaemia
Hypoglycaemia is the greatest danger and more common than hyperglycaemia. This is usually caused by:
- Failure to take food (keeping the patient waiting at lunch time!).
- Overdose of insulin (or drugs, including alcohol).
- Too much exercise.

Hypoglycaemia is of rapid onset, and the sooner treatment is given, the easier, safer and more effective it is (Table 4.3).

Management (Table 4.3)
Never give insulin to treat coma in a diabetic, unless there is absolutely no question that it is caused by hyperglycaemia. Give glucose in all other instances.

Table 4.2   Cardiopulmonary resuscitation

Summon medical assistance

Artificial ventilation

Clear airway of mucus, blood, vomit, etc,
extend neck and hold up chin

Endotracheal intubation if possible *or* Brook
airway

Use positive pressure ventilation, by mouth
to mouth, Ambu bag and airway, or by
machine, inflating 10–12 times each
minute

Give oxygen at 8–10 litres each minute
(adult), slightly less in children

External cardiac massage

Place patient on a firm surface

Press rhythmically on sternum 60 times each
minute, depressing it to 4–5 cm (adult) or
2–3 cm (child)
Record ECG:
If in ventricular fibrillation, defibrillate then
infuse lignocaine 1–4 mg/kg IV

If in asystole, give 5 ml of 1 in 10 000 adrenaline IV to produce ventricular fibrillation:
give 5 ml of 10% calcium chloride or gluconate; then as above

---

Following resuscitation, consider basic cause of arrest, eg haemorrhage, electrolyte distur-
bance or drug toxicity, and treat accordingly. Transfer to ICU or CCU

Remember: Airway, Breathing, Circulation, Drugs.

4.8 Corticosteroid insufficiency (see also Section 3.4)

Many patients are on, or have been treated with, corticosteroids and often
appear healthy. They lack the capacity to respond with the normal
physiological output of endogenous corticosteroids in response to the stress
of:

- operation;
- infection;
- trauma;
- severe vomiting.

Collapse (adrenal crisis) can be precipitated if an adequate steroid 'cover' is
not given in these patients.

Table 4.3 Collapse in a diabetic[a]

	Hypoglycaemia	Hyperglycaemia
Features	Warm sweaty skin Rapid, full pulse Dilated pupils Anxiety or irritability later Confusion and disorientation Rapid onset of coma	Dry skin and mouth Weak rapid pulse. BP↓ Increasing drowsiness (± acetone on breath) Vomiting, hyperventilation Slow decline into coma
Management	Take blood (for glucose level) Immediately give glucose 25 g orally (or 4 sugar lumps or Lucozade) if conscious. If unconscious, immediately give either 50 ml 50% sterile dextrose IV or glucagon 1 mg IM and then oral glucose when patient arouses	Take blood (for glucose level) Put up an IV infusion of 8·4% bicarbonate Obtain medical opinion

[a]There may be other causes

Recognition
Acute adrenal insufficiency may closely resemble a faint, with:
● Collapse
● Weakness
● Nausea (with or without vomiting)
● *But* hypotension that does not respond to lying the patient flat.

Management (Table 4.1)
(1) Lay the patient flat, with the legs raised.
(2) Give 500 mg methylprednisolone (or 200 mg hydrocortisone) IV.
(3) Summon medical assistance.
(4) Take blood for glucose and electrolyte estimation.
(5) Give glucose if there is hypoglycaemia (25 g orally or IV).
(6) Put up an intravenous infusion of normal saline or glucose–saline. Give 1 litre over 2 hours, together with 200 mg hydrocortisone sodium succinate, repeating this at 4–6-hourly intervals as required and monitor the blood pressure.

Determine and deal with the underlying cause when the blood pressure has been stabilised. Control of pain and infection are particularly important and steroid supplementation must be continued for at least 3 days after the blood pressure has returned to normal.

4.9 Epilepsy

A grand mal epileptic convulsive episode is a sequence of

Aura → Tonic phase → Clonic phase → Recovery

Epileptics vary one from another in the frequency and severity of fits and also individually have good and bad 'phases'. Fits may be precipitated by:
- withdrawal of anticonvulsant medication;
- epileptogenic drugs, such as:
  - (a) tricyclics
  - (b) phenothiazines
  - (c) alcohol
  - (d) enflurane
  - (e) methohexitone (and other IV anaesthetics);
- fatigue;
- infection;
- stress;
- starvation or hypoglycaemia;
- menstruation;
- flickering lights.

Management involves protecting the patient from hurting him/herself, and maintaining the airway. Most fits resolve spontaneously within 5 minutes; failing this, treat as status epilepticus (see Table 4.1).

Status epilepticus

Status epilepticus is recurrent seizures, occurring without recovery of consciousness between fits. This involves high mortality and morbidity if not rapidly controlled, especially in the elderly.

Management
(1) Maintain airway and oxygenation.
(2) Control seizures (eg diazepam: 10 mg Diazemuls IV for adults; rectal diazepam for young children).
(3) Treat hyperthermia as required.
(4) Maintain hydration and electrolyte balance.
(5) Treat any obvious cause.
(6) If status epilepticus continues or returns, give chlormethiazole (10·8% solution) at a rate of 60–150 drops per minute in an IV infusion, giving up to 100 ml (up to 800 mg).

4.10 Anaphylaxis

Points to remember:
- Anaphylaxis can follow the use of any drug, particularly penicillin and intravenous anaesthetics.
- Anaphylaxis is more like to occur after the parenteral use of a drug.
- Groups particularly liable to develop anaphylaxis include patients
  - (a) known to be allergic to the particular drug;
  - (b) with any allergies;
  - (c) with asthma, eczema or hay fever.
- Patients may develop an anaphylactic reaction even in the absence of a prior history of allergy to the drug, or even, occasionally, in the absence of any known previous exposure to the drug.
- Anaphylaxis can arise within a couple of minutes, or up to 30 minutes after drug administration.

Recognition
- Collapse
- Acute hypotension
- Wheezing (bronchoconstriction)
- Possibly angioedema and/or urticaria.

Management
(1) Lay patient flat with legs raised.
(2) Give appropriate medication immediately (see Table 4.4).
(3) Maintain the airway.

Prevention
When giving any injection (particularly intramuscularly), have the patient lying flat; he/she is then unlikely to faint. If the injection is given to the standing patient, there may be a delay in distinguishing anaphylaxis from a simple faint. Furthermore, collapsing patients can damage themselves as they fall.

4.11 Psychiatric emergencies

A psychiatric emergency generates tensions among staff and relatives, and often leads to a crisis out of proportion to the patient's clinical state. First of all, try to make contact with the patient. A disturbed person is often incorrectly treated, as if he or she had no intelligence or awareness of his or her surroundings. Such patients may well comprehend what is being said to them, even though they cannot respond. Do not press questions, but

Table 4.4   Drug treatment of anaphylaxis

	Comments	Route	Dose
Adrenaline injection	1 in 1000 solution used (contains 1 mg/ml) Give IM rather than subcutaneously	IM	0·5–1·0 ml of a 1 in 1000 solution
Methylprednisolone (Solumedrone)	This is effective more rapidly than hydrocortisone but is more expensive. Is already in solution	IV	500 mg
or Hydrocortisone	Only advantage of hydrocortisone sodium phosphate (Ef Cortelan) over sodium succinate (eg Solu-Cortef) is that phosphate is already in solution Hydrocortisone sodium phosphate may cause transient paraesthesia after IV injection Effect quicker by IV than IM use, but still takes 2–4 hours (persists 8 hours)	IV	100–500 mg slowly

offer an explanation of the situation. Tell the patient where he/she is and what is happening.

Where possible, call the duty psychiatrist. The acutely disturbed patient calls for decisive action, but with the mute, amnesic, withdrawn or depressed patient there is less urgency.

Most mentally ill patients can be persuaded to accept help voluntarily. If the patient is considered a danger to him/herself or others and refuses help, compulsory detention in hospital is required (sectioning) (see Tables 4.5 and 4.6.)

Management of psychiatric emergencies

Actively suicidal patients
- Initiate compulsory detention procedures: admit to hospital.
- Talk to the patient reassuringly.
- If an in-patient might try to leave hospital, take away his/her clothes (and explain why).
- Arrange continual supervision.
- Do not interfere physically if possible.

Acute drug intoxication or drug withdrawal reaction
- If related to cocaine or heroin, call the psychiatrist immediately.
- Take blood and urine (for analysis).
- If related to barbiturate withdrawal, give amylobarbitone 200 mg orally, 8-hourly.
- In other causes, give diazepam 10–30 mg (10 mg slow IV Diazemuls) or chlorpromazine 50–200 mg (orally if possible).
- Admit to hospital.

Delirium tremens
- Consider the possibility that accident, illness or other drugs, rather than alcohol withdrawal, may be responsible.
- Give chlormethiazole 500–1000 mg orally six-hourly initially, then decreasing, or diazepam 5–20 mg IV, or chlordiazepoxide 5–20 mg orally 6-hourly.
- Constantly observe the patient, as chlormethiazole can cause respiratory depression.
- Give Parentrovite IM or IV.
- Admit to hospital.

Acute psychosis
- Take blood and urine (for analysis).
- In panic states, give diazepam 5–20 mg IV (Diazemuls).
- In psychoses or violent drunkenness, give chlorpromazine 25–50 mg IM.
- Initiate compulsory detention procedures; admit to hospital.

Acute depression
- Give diazepam 10 mg orally three times daily or sedate with diazepam 5–20 mg IV (Diazemuls) if very agitated.
- Do not give antidepressants as emergency treatment.
- Admit to hospital.

Disoriented elderly patient
- Ask a close relative to stay with the patient.
- Stop all sedatives.
- Do *not* isolate the patient.
- Admit to hospital.

Compulsory admission or detention of patients
The Mental Health Act 1983 and the Mental Health Act (Scotland) 1960 (Tables 4.5 and 4.6) give powers for admission or detention of people in hospital against their will, if the following conditions apply:

Table 4.5 Compulsory procedures (Mental Health Act 1983) for management of patients with psychiatric disease[a]

Section	Purpose	Duration	Persons making application	Medical recommendations
2	Hospital admission for observation	28 days	Nearest relative or authorised social worker	Both (1) registered medical practitioner and (2) recognised psychiatrist
3	Hospital admission for treatment	One year. May be renewed if appropriate. Patient may appeal to a Mental Health Tribunal in the first 6 months	Nearest relative or authorised social worker (the latter must, where practicable, first consult the nearest relative)	Both (1) registered medical practitioner who knows patient and (2) recognised psychiatrist
4	Hospital admission for observation in emergency (when only one doctor is available and the degree of urgency does not permit delay to obtain a second medical opinion)	72 hours	Any relative or authorised social worker	Registered medical practitioner
5	Emergency detention of an informal patient already in hospital	3 days beginning on the day on which report is furnished		The responsible consultant psychiatrist in charge of the case. His deputy may act on his direct instructions

Table 4.5 Compulsory procedures (Mental Health Act 1983) for management of patients with psychiatric disease[a]—*contd*

Section	Purpose	Duration	Persons making application	Medical recommendations
136	Removal by police to a place of safety. Persons who appear to be mentally disordered in a place to which the public have access, if in immediate need of care or control, may be taken by police to a place of safety to await examination by a doctor and authorised social worker	72 hours	Police officer	

[a]Call the Duty Psychiatrist.

Table 4.6 Compulsory procedures (Mental Health Act Scotland 1960) for management of patients with psychiatric disease[a]

Section	Purpose	Duration	Persons making application	Medical recommendations
24	Hospital admission for observation	28 days	Nearest relative or authorised social worker	Both (1) registered medical practitioner and (2) medical practitioner recognised under s. 27
31	Hospital admission for observation in emergency (where s. 24 is not applicable) *or* Emergency detention of an informal patient already in hospital	7 days	Any relative or authorised social worker	Registered medical practitioner who has examined the patient on that day
104	Removal by police to a place of safety	72 hours	Police officer	

[a] Call the Duty Psychiatrist.

(a) That this patient is suffering from mental disorder of a nature or degree which warrants his/her detention in a hospital under observation for at least a limited period;

(b) That this patient ought to be so detained
  (i) in the interest of the patient's own health or safety, and/or
  (ii) with a view to the protection of other persons;

(c) That informal admission is not appropriate in the circumstances of the case.

To implement the Act, an application and/or medical recommendation has to be made on the appropriate form(s), which completed forms must be lodged with the hospital managers (during working hours the Hospital Secretary, after hours the Nursing Officer in charge or other specified persons) before any order becomes legally valid.

4.12 Chest pain

Angina
Give glyceryl trinitrate 500 µg tablet sublingually or 400 µg spray. Isosorbide dinitrate 5 mg sublingually or nifedipine 5 mg capsule to be bitten are alternatives.

Myocardial infarction
Give diamorphine 5 mg IM or IV as analgesic plus 12·5 mg prochlorperazine IM as anti-emetic. Call for medical assistance immediately. Give oxygen if the patient is breathless. Lie the patient flat only if he or she is hypotensive.

5

Therapeutics

This chapter is not intended to be totally comprehensive, and alternative therapies may well be available. The following points should be borne in mind: (1) Drug doses should be modified as necessary in children, the elderly and in various disease states (see below); (2) The term 'contra-indication' in this chapter often refers only to a relative contra-indication; (3) Drug interactions and adverse reactions noted herein are not always frequent or of great clinical significance; (4) Always check drug doses, contra-indications, interactions and adverse reactions in the latest edition of the *British National Formulary*, the *Dental Practitioners' Formulary* (UK), or the *Physicians Desk Reference* (USA); (5) Prescribe only drugs with which you are totally familiar.

5.1 Prescribing

The Prescribers' Journal (Department of Health), the *Adverse Reaction Bulletin*, *Monthly Index of Medical Specialities (MIMS)*, and the *Drug and Therapeutics Bulletin* (the Consumers' Association), also contain helpful information concerning recent advances and other aspects of prescribing, including guidance on economy and the relative value of drugs.

Points to remember:

● Write drug names in full, in ink.

● Use non-proprietary drug titles whenever possible.

● Drug dosage may need modification for use in children, the elderly and in patients with various diseases or on certain drugs (Tables 5.22–5.24). Where possible, drugs should be avoided in pregnancy (Section 3.10).

● The strength or quantity to be contained in capsules, lozenges, tablets, etc, should be stated by the prescriber.

● Containers are usually labelled with the name of the preparation and strength.

Prescribing drugs in hospitals

Fully and provisionally registered medical and hospital dental staff are authorised to prescribe drugs for in-patients, patients being discharged, and out-patients (except heroin and cocaine for addicts). However, unregistered locum staff or students do not have authority to prescribe drugs, so that prescriptions written by unregistered staff must be authorised (ie signed) by a provisionally or fully registered doctor or dentist. Drugs may be given when required, at the discretion of nursing staff. Nurses should not be expected to take responsibility for choosing from a selection of prescriptions for similar drugs, different routes of administration and doses, without the prescriber specifying the criteria to be considered when making such decisions. It is reasonable to expect nurses to recognise night sedatives, analgesics and anti-emetics, but where 'when required' drugs are prescribed for other indications, these should be clearly stated in writing.

Nurses trained and authorised by the authorities to give IV drugs may do so, provided that this does not require them to make entry into a vein; in other words, they can give drugs into a 'drip'. The first dose should be given by the dental surgeon, who can then check for adverse reactions.

In the UK, heroin and cocaine for addicts may only be prescribed by practitioners specially licensed by the Secretary of State. If an addict is admitted, the house officer should contact one of the licensed psychiatrists for heroin or cocaine to be given. This restriction applies only to the prescribing of heroin and cocaine for addicts and places no restriction on prescribing these drugs for the relief of pain due to organic disease or injury. However, morphine sulphate is preferred for the treatment of very severe pain (Section 5.5), unless there is a head injury or respiratory disease.

Prescribing drugs in practice

Drugs in the DPF can be prescribed by a dental practitioner on form FP14 (England and Wales) or GP14 (Scotland), as a charge to the NHS. Other drugs can be prescribed privately.

Drugs and food absorption

The following oral drugs should be given at least 30 minutes *before* food:

- Erythromycin
- Rifampicin
- Penicillins
- Tetracyclines (except doxycycline)

The absorption of aspirin and paracetamol may also be delayed by food. Most other oral drugs are best given with or after food

Table 5.1   Rough guide for prescribing for children

Age of child (years)	Percentage of adult drug dose
1	25
6	50
12	75

Prescribing for children (see also Tables 5.1 and 5.2)

● Some drugs (eg, tetracyclines) are contra-indicated under the age of 7–8 years.

● Some drugs (eg diazepam) may have anomalous effects.

● Oral preparations are invariably preferable to injectable drugs.

● Doses of all drugs are much lower than for adults. As a rough guide, Tables 5.1 and 5.2 can be used, but always check against the recommended dose per unit body weight.

Prescribing in pregnancy and during breast feeding (see also Section 3.10, Table 3.22 and Tables 5.22–5.24)
Because of the danger of damage to the foetus, all drugs should be avoided in pregnancy, unless their use is essential. Tetracyclines, in particular, should be avoided.

Prescribing for the elderly (see also Tables 5.22–5.24)
When prescribing for the elderly, drug doses are almost invariably lower.

Table 5.2   Prescribing for children

| Age | Average weight | | Drug dose | |
	(kg)	(lb)	as percentage of adult dose	in mg/kg if adult dose = 1·0 mg/kg
Over 2 weeks	3·2	7	12	2·0
4 months	6·5	14	20	2·0
1 year	10·0	22	25	
3 years	15·0	33	33	1·5
7 years	23	51	50	
12 years	37	82	75	1·25

Compliance may be poor, and care should be taken when there is the possibility of renal or hepatic dysfunction; this will necessitate reduced doses.

5.2 Giving an intramuscular injection

Antimicrobials and various other drugs (eg corticosteroids, iron preparations, diazepam) may be given intramuscularly (IM). The indications for IM antimicrobials in dentistry have been reduced somewhat since the advent of oral amoxycillin, which gives extremely high blood levels within 1–2 hours, and persists for 9–10 hours. Patient compliance is increased with the use of this drug.

For all IM (or any other) injections, it is wise to have the patient lying down beforehand, in case he or she faints. If the patient collapses while having an injection when standing, there is the possibility of injury, and you may have a few moments of anxiety trying to differentiate a simple faint from anaphylaxis.

If an IM injection is definitely indicated, check that:

● The patient is not allergic to the drug or that the drug is otherwise contra-indicated.
● The expiry date of the drug has not passed.
● The correct drug (and solvent) is used; this is particularly important if another person (eg a nurse) makes up the drug.

Site of injection
The anterolateral aspect of the thigh is the preferred site (fig. 5.1).

Method of injection
The following procedures should be carried out when giving an IM injection:

(1) The patient should be lying down.
(2) Swab the site with isopropyl alcohol.
(3) Allow the area to dry.
(4) Rapidly pierce the skin and muscle with the needle (size 19 or 20 for large volumes of fluid, size 21 or 23 for small volumes).
(5) Aspirate to ensure needle is not in a blood vessel.
(6) Inject slowly.
(7) Withdraw the needle and swab the area.
(8) Observe the patient for adverse reactions (30 minutes in the case of antimicrobials).

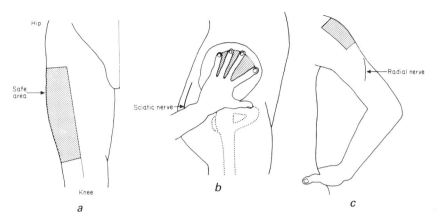

Fig. 5.1   Sites for intramuscular injection.

(*a*) *Antero-lateral aspect of the thigh. The best site.* Larger injections may be given into the vastus lateralis muscle on the antero-lateral aspect of the thigh, where there is a large mass of muscle free from important vessels or nerves.

(*b*) *Anterior part of the upper and outer quadrant of the buttock.* To find the safest place for an intramuscular injection into the right buttock, place the tip of the left index finger on the anterior superior iliac spine and the tip of the middle finger, abducted as shown in the diagram, just below iliac crest. The injection site is then into the gluteal muscles within the triangle formed by the fingers and the iliac crest. *Do not inject into* the 'bottom', as there is a danger of damage to the sciatic nerve.

(*c*) *Outer aspect of the shoulder.* Small injections can be given into the deltoid muscles on the outer aspect of the shoulder. The shirt or blouse must be removed so that you will not inject too low, since there is a danger of damage to the radial nerve.

5.3 Management of common oral disorders

Management of common acute oral disorders is outlined in Table 5.3; management of other oral disorders is outlined in Table 5.4.

Table 5.3   Management of the more common acute oral problems

Disorder	Management
Acute pulpitis	Open tooth (or extract); extirpate pulp (arrange endodontics); analgesia
Acute apical periodontitis	Open tooth for drainage and relieve occlusion (or extract); ± antimicrobials[a]; analgesia
Acute apical abscess	Incise and drain if pointing *or* open tooth for drainage and relieve occlusion (or extract); ± antimicrobials[a,b]; analgesia

Table 5.3   Management of the more common acute oral problems—*contd*

Disorder	Management
Acute pericoronitis	Relieve or extract opposing tooth if traumatising operculum; caustics to operculum ± antimicrobials[b] (if recurrent arrange extraction); ± hot saline mouth baths
Acute ulcerative gingivitis	Oral debridement; mouthwashes of hydrogen peroxide; antimicrobial,[c] arrange periodontal care
Lateral periodontal abscess	± extraction or antimicrobials; hot saline mouth baths; analgesia
Acute bacterial sialadenitis	Determine cause (usually duct obstruction or xerostomia); antimicrobials (flucloxacillin); ± drainage
Acute fascial space infections	Drain if possible; high dose antimicrobials;[b] admit patients with Ludwig's angina
Acute candidosis	Determine cause; antifungals (nystatin or amphotericin or miconazole; Section 5.7)
Acute viral stomatitis	Symptomatic treatment mainly is available: (*a*) Reduce fever; give paracetamol elixir (*b*) Analgesia (as above in (*a*)) (*c*) Maintain fluid intake (*d*) Sedation if required (promethazine) (*e*) Maintain oral hygiene (mouthwashes of chlorhexidine 0·2%) (*f*) Soft diet (*g*) ± antivirals, eg acyclovir (particularly useful in the immunocompromised patient) for herpetic infections (Section 5.7)

Acute sinusitis (also for oro-antral fistula)	(*a*) Inhalations
	      Steam ±
	      Ephedrine hydrochloride nasal drops 1% (not in patients on monoamine oxidase inhibitors)
	      or oxymetazoline *or*
	      aromatic mixtures such as Karvol (menthol, chlorbutol, cinnamon oil, pine oil, thymol and terpineol) *or*
	      menthol and benzoin, *or*
	      menthol and eucalyptus, *or*
	      tinct. benzoin Co.
	(*b*) Antimicrobials
	      Amoxycillin, erythromycin *or* co-trimoxazole
	(c) Analgesia

Dry socket	See Section 7.7

[a] A penicillin if there are no contra-indications to this (see Section 5.7)
[b] Penicillin *or* metronidazole are indicated if there are systemic effects, pyrexia, trismus or severe lymphadenitis.
[c] Penicillin or metronidazole.

5.4 Cryosurgery and laser surgery

Cryosurgery

Indications

Some patients with intractable facial pain (use cryoanalgesia), leukoplakias (keratosis), mucous extravasation cysts, small haemangiomas, palliation in severe erosive lesions, or palliation in malignant neoplasia. The diagnosis should be established by histology in leukoplakias and mucous extravasation cysts.

Procedure

The probes are usually either nitrous oxide or liquid nitrogen. Nitrous oxide is prone to breakdown, so cylinders and a scavenging system are needed. Liquid nitrogen is perhaps better than the nitrous oxide type, but requires large volumes of liquid nitrogen.

Dosage in cryosurgery is largely empirical at present, but nitrous oxide cryoprobes are usually applied for periods of 30 seconds or one minute, and very often multiple freezes are employed, with thawing between each freeze to maximise the tissue damage that occurs secondary to ice recrystallisation and hypertonicity. One of the principal advantages of cryosurgery is the minimal scarring produced. However, liquid nitrogen probes and sprays are quite capable of full-thickness skin necrosis, and dosage is therefore usually limited to 15- or 30-second applications when the cosmetic result is an important consideration. The temperature gradients and lowest temperatures achieved using liquid nitrogen make this refrigerant particularly useful in the management of neoplastic conditions and recalcitrant lesions such as keloid scars, and several 1- or 2-minute freezes may be necessary in these conditions.

Laser surgery

Indications

Although laser surgery is expensive, potentially hazardous and may possibly be followed by malignant changes in some precancerous lesions, it is used in some centres for the treatment of leukoplakia, early neoplasia and orofacial haemangiomas, particularly those affecting the floor of the mouth. As in cryosurgery, histopathological diagnosis should be obtained preoperatively. Treatment is usually only possible under general anaesthesia.

Procedure

The carbon dioxide laser is most commonly used in intra-oral laser therapy. This is a cutting laser. It is essential to follow laser safety

Table 5.4 Management of other oral disorders

Disorder	Relieve any precipitating factors	Topical corticosteroids if symptomatic	Intra-lesional steroid	Systemic steroids	Others
Actinomycosis	–	–	–	–	Amoxycillin or tetracycline
Angioedema allergic	Avoid allergen	–	–	If airway threatened	Antihistamines
hereditary	Avoid trauma	–	–	–	Stanozolol
Angular stomatitis	Treat denture stomatitis	–	–	–	Miconazole
Aphthae	+	+	±	–	Tetracycline or other mouthwashes sometimes
Atypical facial pain	–	–	–	–	Antidepressants
Behçet's syndrome	–	+	±	±	Colchicine
Bell's palsy	–	–	–	+	Protect cornea
Burning mouth syndrome	+	–	–	–	Sometimes antidepressants
Candidosis acute	+	–	–	–	Antifungal
denture stomatitis	+	–	–	–	Antifungal + leave denture out of mouth at night
Crohn's disease	–	–	+	±	Salazopyrine. Correct nutritional defects
Cytotoxic-induced ulcers	–	–	–	–	Symptomatic ± folinic acid
Dermatitis herpetiformis	Gluten-free diet	–	–	–	Dapsone
Desquamative gingivitis	Oral hygiene	+	–	–	Dapsone sometimes
Dry mouth	Avoid drugs and smoking	–	–	–	Saliva substitute. Treat any candidosis; fluorides

Table 5.4 Management of other oral disorders—*contd*

Disorder	Relieve any precipitating factors	Topical corticosteroids if symptomatic	Intra-lesional steroid	Systemic steroid	Others
Erythema migrans	Some foods	–	–	–	–
Erythema multiforme	Drugs, infections	–	–	±	Acyclovir if herpes-induced
Epidermolysis bullosa	Avoid trauma	–	–	–	Phenytoin. Vitamin E
Fibrous dysplasia		–	–	–	Excise
Giant cell arteritis		–	–	+	Medical advice
Glossitis (see vitamin deficiency)					
Hairy leukoplakia		–	–	–	Acyclovir/etretinate/Zidovudine possibly. Refer to AIDS physician
Herpes simplex stomatitis		–	–	–	Acyclovir if seen early or immunocompromised.
recurrence	UV light		–	–	As above. Also uvistat in sunbathing.
Herpes zoster		–	–	±	Analgesics. Protect cornea. Acyclovir
Herpangina/Hand, foot and mouth disease		–	–	–	Symptomatic
Infectious mononucleosis		–	–	–	Steroids if faucial oedema threatens airway
Kaposi's sarcoma (in AIDS)		–	–	–	Refer to AIDS physician
Keratoses	Trauma, smoking	–	–	–	Excise: cryosurgery Etretinate in some

Table 5.4 Management of other oral disorders—*contd*

Disorder	Relieve any precipitating factors	Topical corticosteroids if symptomatic	Intra-lesional steroid	Systemic steroid	Others
Lichen planus					
non-erosive	Drugs	+	−	−	−
erosive	Drugs	+	±	−	Therapy depends on severity. Etretinate may help
Linear IgA disease	−	−	−	−	Dapsone
Migraine	Stress, some foods	−	−	−	Propranolol prophylaxis Ergotamine
Migranous neuralgia	Alcohol	−	−	−	Propranolol prophylaxis Ergotamine
Mumps	−	−	−	−	Symptomatic
Neoplasms					
benign	Trauma	−	−	−	Excise
malignant	Smoking Trauma	−	−	−	Surgery ± radiotherapy dependent on diagnosis
Paget's disease	−	−	−	−	Diphosphonates ± calcitonin
Pemphigoid	Drugs rarely	+	−	±	Systemic steroids if severe disease or skin/other mucosae involved
Pemphigus	Drugs rarely	−	−	+	Plus azathioprine or gold for steroid-sparing
Pigmented localised lesions	−	−	−	−	Excise usually
Radiation mucositis	Oral hygiene	−	−	−	Symptomatic. Topical steroids for prophylaxis
Sarcoidosis	−	−	−	±	Systemic steroids if eyes involved

Table 5.4 Management of other oral disorders—*contd*

Disorder	Relieve any precipitating factors	Topical corticosteroids if symptomatic	Intra-lesional steroid	Systemic steroids	Others
Sialosis	Alcoholism Diabetes	–	–	–	–
Sjögren's syndrome		–	–	–	Saliva substitute. Treat infections. Fluorides
Submucous fibrosis	Areca nut	–	+	–	Surgery if severe restriction of mouth opening
Syphilis	–	–	–	–	Penicillin
Taste disturbances	Infections, systemic disease	–	–	–	Oral hygiene
TMJ pain-dysfunction	Stress, para-function	–	–	–	Possibly antidepressants. Possibly occlusal adjustments
Toxoplasmosis	–	–	–	–	Sulphonamide + pyrimethamine
Traumatic ulcers	+	+	–	–	Symptomatic usually
Trigeminal neuralgia	Avoid trigger zone	–	–	–	Carbamazepine (or phenytoin). May need surgery if unresponsive
Tuberculosis	–	–	–	–	Antibiotics: rifampicin, isoniazid, ethambutol, streptomycin
Vitamin deficiency	GI disease	–	–	–	Correct deficiency
White sponge naevus	–	–	–	–	–

recommendations and use non-inflammable anaesthetic agents and to avoid reflections from surgical instruments. Adequate access and attention to operator comfort will allow prolonged and precise vaporisation of tissue. Haemostasis occurs during vaporisation, secondary to coagulation of small vessels in the wound-bed, and tumour seeding is therefore usually prevented.

Laser therapy can be carried out under microscopic or endoscopic control, and may be followed by less pain and swelling than that which normally follows surgical excision or cryotherapy.

Potential hazards of laser therapy include damage to the eyes and other tissues as a result of reflection of the laser beam from surgical retractors, mouth-props, or anaesthetic tube couplings, and vaporisation of anaesthetic tubes, leading to ignition of flammable anaesthetic agents. Regular servicing of equipment is important, and, ideally, should be carried out in the operating theatre where the treatment takes place.

5.5 Analgesics, narcotics and drug abuse (see also Table 5.5, 5.22–5.24)

General principles for the use of analgesics

- Where possible, treat the cause of pain.
- Relieve factors which lower the pain threshold (fatigue, anxiety, depression).
- Chronic pain requires regular analgesia (not just 'as required').
- Try simple analgesics initially, before embarking on more potent preparations; avoid polypharmacy (Table 5.5).
- Aspirin has long been in use, and the efficacy and adverse effects are well recognised. The same comments cannot be said to apply to all of the newer analgesics.
- Avoid aspirin in children under the age of 12 years and mothers who are breast-feeding (possible association with Reye's syndrome — a serious liver disease) and in patients with gastric disease or a bleeding tendency (Table 5.16). Paracetamol is preferred in these instances.
- Aspirin is only one of the group of non-steroidal anti-inflammatory drugs (NSAIDS). Most NSAIDS can cause peptic ulceration and further deterioration of renal function, if this is already impaired. NSAIDS may also worsen asthma and cause fluid retention as well as nausea, diarrhoea or tinnitus. NSAIDS also increase methotrexate toxicity, and interfere with antihypertensives and diuretics.

- Opiates are contra-indicated in patients with head injury, since they interfere with pupillary responses (Table 5.22) and suppress respiration.
- Many of the more potent analgesics (including pentazocine and distalgesic) produce dependence and are now used less frequently.

Opioids, narcotics and drug addiction (Table 5.5)

Opioids are analgesics used for moderate to severe pain. They may cause dependence, constipation, respiratory depression, nausea, drowsiness and urinary retention. They are generally contra-indicated in patients with head injuries, liver or kidney disease, those who are pregnant, or breast feeding, and those taking monoamine oxidase inhibitors (see also Tables 5.22–5.24).

Narcotics are 'Controlled Drugs', all capable of causing addiction and include:

- Dextromoramide (5 and 10 mg tablets).
- Dipipanone (10 mg tablets with 30 mg cyclizine hydrochloride as Diconal).
- Methadone (5 mg tablets). Beware methadone in the elderly or debilitated patient, as accumulation occurs.
- Phenazocine (5 mg tablets).
- Pethidine (50–100 mg SC or IM). This drug is less potent than morphine, but has similar side-effects. It is less likely than morphine to cause ileus in post-operative patients.
- Morphine (10–20 mg IM, or 5–10 mg IV, slowly). Oral preparations include:
  - (a) Nepenthe 8·4 mg/ml) and papaveretum (20 mg/ml). Often causes hypotension, vomiting, respiratory depression, and excessive sedation.
  - (b) Diamorphine or heroin (5 mg orally, or 2·5 mg IM or IV, slowly). Causes less hypotension and vomiting than morphine. Highly addictive. Also effective on oral administration.
  - (c) Piritramide (20 mg IM) is effective for post-operative analgesia, but is more sedating than morphine.
  - (d) Fentanyl (100–200 µg IV or IM) is potent, but may cause bradycardia, hypertension or nausea with respiratory depression.

Drug addiction is increasingly common, particularly in urban areas such as the 'new towns'. The most serious problems in the management of addicts, whether because of alcohol or drugs, are overdosage, withdrawal effects, behavioural problems (including theft), and violence. Hepatitis and

Table 5.5 Analgesics (see also Tables 5.22–5.24 and Table 7.2)[a]

Analgesic	Comments	Tablet contains	Route	Adult dose
Aspirin	Mild analgesic: an NSAID Causes gastric irritation Interferes with haemostasis Contra-indicated in bleeding disorders, children, asthma, late pregnancy, peptic ulcers, renal disease	300 mg	O	300–600 mg up to 6 times a day after meals (use *soluble* or *dispersible* or *enteric-coated* aspirin) (Maximum 4 g daily)
Mefenamic acid	Mild analgesic: an NSAID May be contra-indicated in asthma, gastro-intestinal, renal and liver disease, and pregnancy May cause diarrhoea or haemolytic anaemia	250 mg *or* 500 mg	O	250–500 mg up to 3 times a day
Diflunisal	Analgesic for mild to moderate pain: an NSAID Long action: twice a day dose only. Effective against pain from bone and joint Contra-indicated in pregnancy, peptic ulcer, allergies, renal and liver disease	250 mg *or* 500 mg	O	250–500 mg twice a day
Paracetamol	Mild analgesic: not usually termed an NSAID Hepatotoxic in overdose or prolonged use Contra-indicated in liver or renal disease or those on zidovudine	500 mg	O	500–1000 mg up to 6 times a day (maximum 4 g daily)
Codeine phosphate*	Analgesic for moderate pain Contra-indicated in late pregnancy and liver disease. Avoid alcohol May cause sedation and constipation Reduces cough reflex	15 mg *or* 30 mg	O	10–60 mg up to 6 times a day (or 30 mg IM)

Table 5.5 Analgesics (see also Tables 5.22–5.24 and Table 7.2)^a—contd

Analgesic	Comments	Tablet contains	Route	Adult dose
Dextropropoxyphene*	Analgesic for moderate pain Risk of respiratory depression in overdose, especially if taken with alcohol May cause dependence Occasional hepatotoxicity No more effective as an analgesic than paracetamol or aspirin alone	65 mg	O	65 mg up to 4 times a day
Dihydrocodeine tartrate*	Analgesic for moderate pain May cause nausea, drowsiness and constipation Contra-indicated in children, hypothyroidism, asthma, renal disease May increase post-op. dental pain	30 mg	O	30 mg up to 4 times a day (or 50 mg IM)
Pentazocine*	Analgesic for moderate pain May produce dependence May produce hallucinations May provoke withdrawal symptoms in narcotic addicts Contra-indicated in pregnancy, children, hypertension, respiratory depression, head injuries or raised intracranial pressure. There is a low risk of dependence	25 mg	O	50 mg up to 4 times a day (or 30 mg IM or IV)
Buprenorphine*	Potent analgesic More potent analgesic than pentazocine, longer action than morphine No hallucinations May cause salivation, sweating, dizziness and vomiting	0·2 mg	Sublingual	0·2–0·4 mg up to 4 times a day (or 0·3 mg IM)

Table 5.5 Analgesics (see also Tables 5.22–5.24 and Table 7.2)[a]—contd

Analgesic	Comments	Tablet contains	Route	Adult dose
Buprenorphine* (contd)	Respiratory depression in overdose. Can cause dependence Contra-indicated in children, pregnancy, MAOI, liver disease or respiratory disease			
Meptazinol*	Potent analgesic Claimed to have a low incidence of respiratory depression. Side-effects as buprenorphine	No tablet	IM or IV	75–100 mg up to 6 times a day
Phenazocine*	Analgesic for severe pain May cause nausea	5 mg	O or sublingual	5 mg up to 4 times a day
Pethidine*	Potent analgesic Less potent than morphine Contra-indicated in MAOI Risk of dependence	No tablet	SC or IM	25–100 mg up to 4 times a day
Morphine*	Potent analgesic Often causes nausea and vomiting. Reduces cough reflex, causes pupil constriction Risk of dependence	See BNF	SC or IM or O or suppository	5–10 mg
Diamorphine*	Potent analgesic More potent than pethidine and morphine but more euphoria and dependence	10 mg	SC or IM or O	2–5 mg by injection; 5–10 mg orally

[a]There are many NSAIDS
*Opioids

AIDS, as well as other infections, are increasingly common, particularly among intravenous drug misusers. Disturbed behaviour in a drug addict may be caused by withdrawal symptoms and the patient may need compulsory detention (see Section 4.11). Addicts in need of a 'fix' will often falsely complain of severe pain or injury.

5.6 Antidepressants (see Tables 5.6 and 5.7 and also Tables 5.22–5.24)

General principles for the use of antidepressants

● In addition to drugs for the treatment of depression, psychotherapy and possibly physical treatment are required.

● If there is any possibility of a suicide attempt, the patient must be seen by a psychiatrist as a matter of urgency (Section 4.11).

● There may be an interval as long as 3 – 4 weeks before the antidepressant action takes place. Monitoring of plasma concentrations of the drug may be helpful in ensuring optimal dosage.

● Prescribe only limited amounts of antidepressants, as there is a danger that the patient may use them in a suicide attempt.

Table 5.6 Antidepressants

Tricyclics and tetracyclics	Monoamine oxidase inhibitors (MAOI)
Use with caution in	**Use with caution in**
Cardiovascular disease	Cardiovascular disease
Epilepsy	Epilepsy
Liver disease	Liver disease
Diabetes	Phaeochromocytoma
Hypertension	
Glaucoma	
Mania	
Urinary retention	
Prostatic hypertrophy	
May interact with	**May interact with**
Barbiturates	Barbiturates
MAOI	Some sympathomimetic amines
Antihypertensives	Tricyclics
General anaesthetics	Narcotics
	Antihypertensives
	Foods such as some meat or yeast extracts, cheese, wine

Note: Neither group significantly interacts with lignocaine, prilocaine or the doses of adrenaline found in dental LA. Either group may cause or worsen xerostomia.

Table 5.7   Some other antidepressants

	Comments (see also Table 5.6 and Section 5.16 and 5.20)	Preparation contains	Route	Dose
Amitriptyline	Tricyclic Antidepressant effect may not be seen until up to 30 days after start Sedative effect also When treatment established, use single dose at night Contra-indicated after recent myocardial infarction	25 mg or 50 mg	O	25–75 mg daily in divided dose
Dothiepin	Tricyclic Anxiolytic effect also useful in atypical facial pain When treatment established, use single dose at night	25 mg or 75 mg	O	25 mg three times a day or 75 mg at night
Clomipramine	Tricyclic Equally as effective as amitriptyline but less sedative effect Useful in phobic or obsessional states	10 mg or 25 mg	O	10–100 mg daily in divided doses
Flupenthixol	Not a tricyclic or MAOI Fewer side-effects Contra-indicated in cardiovascular, hepatic or renal disease, Parkinsonism, or excitable or overactive patients	0·5 mg or 1 mg	O	1–3 mg daily in morning

● The natural history of depression is of remission after 3 – 12 months. Do not withdraw antidepressants prematurely.

● Doses should be reduced for the elderly patient.

● Antidepressants often cause a dry mouth, but the complaint of dry mouth may also be a manifestation of depression.

● Tricyclic antidepressants interact with noradrenaline, but not significantly with the adrenaline in dental local anaesthetic solutions.

● Monoamine oxidase inhibitors (MAOI) do not significantly interact with adrenaline in dental local anaesthetic solutions.

5.7 Antimicrobials in dentistry (see also Tables 5.22–5.24)

Antimicrobials will not remove pus; drainage is therefore essential.

Indications (see Tables 5.3 and 5.4)

Infections (together with appropriate surgical or other measures)
- Infections of fascial spaces of the neck.
- Osteomyelitis.
- Odontogenic infections in ill or toxic patients (eg immunocompromised).
- Acute ulcerative gingivitis.

Prophylaxis
- Of infective endocarditis (Section 3.3).
- In cerebrospinal rhinorrhoea.
- In facial fractures or compound skull fractures.
- In major oral and maxillofacial surgery (eg osteotomies or tumour resection).
- In surgery in immunocompromised or debilitated patients, or following radiotherapy to the jaws.
- Possibly in patients with ventriculo-atrial shunts and prosthetic hip replacements (Section 3.14).

Other
Indicated in some instances of:
- Pericoronitis.
- Dental abscess.
- Dry socket.
- Minor oral surgery.

Choice of antimicrobial

The bacteria which cause most odontogenic infections are sensitive to penicillins. Anaerobes have now been implicated in many odontogenic infections, and these often respond to penicillins or metronidazole. Very high blood antimicrobial levels can now be achieved with oral amoxycillin, with good patient compliance (see below and Tables 5.8 and 5.9).

Pus (as much as possible) should be sent for culture and sensitivities, but antimicrobials should be started immediately if they are indicated. Use another antimicrobial if the patient has had penicillin within the previous month (resistant bacteria).

Table 5.8   Some antibacterials (see also Tables 5.22–5.24)

	Comments	Route	Dose
Penicillins	Most oral bacterial infections respond to penicillin. Oral phenoxymethyl penicillin is usually effective and is cheap. Amoxycillin is often used and is usually effective, but almost four times as expensive		
Amoxycillin	Orally active (absorption better than ampicillin) Broad spectrum penicillin derivative *Staphylococcus aureus* often resistant Not resistant to penicillinase Contra-indicated in penicillin-hypersensitivity Rashes in infectious mononucleosis, cytomegalovirus infection, lymphoid leukaemia, lymphoma, allopurinol May cause diarrhoea	O, IM or IV	250–500 mg 8-hourly (see Table 3.7) about endocarditis)
Augmentin (trade name)	Mixture of amoxycillin and potassium clavulanate (inhibits some penicillinases and therefore is active against most *Staph. aureus*; inhibits some lactamases and is therefore active against some Gram-negative and penicillin-resistant bacteria) Contra-indicated in penicillin-hypersensitivity	O	1 tablet 8-hourly
Ampicillin	Less oral absorption than amoxycillin Otherwise as for amoxycillin. (There are many analogues but these have few, if any, advantages) Contra-indicated in penicillin-hypersensitivity	O, IM or IV	250–500 mg 6-hourly
Benzylpenicillin	Not orally active Most effective penicillin where organism sensitive Not resistant to penicillinase Contra-indicated in penicillin-hypersensitivity Large doses may cause K^+ to fall, Na^+ to rise	IM or IV	300–600 mg 6-hourly
Flucloxacillin	Orally active penicillin derivative Effective against most but not all penicillin-resistant staphylococci (most staphylococci) Contra-indicated in penicillin-hypersensitivity	O or IM	250 mg 6-hourly

Table 5.8 Some antibacterials (see also Tables 5.22–5.24)—*contd*

	Comments	Route	Dose
Phenoxymethyl penicillin (penicillin V)	Orally active Best taken on an empty stomach Not resistant to penicillinase Contra-indicated in penicillin-hypersensitivity	O	250–500 mg 6-hourly
Procaine penicillin	Depot penicillin Not resistant to penicillinase Contra-indicated in penicillin-hypersensitivity Rarely psychotic reaction	IM	300 000 units every 12 hours
Triplopen (trade name)	Depot penicillin Contains benzyl (300 mg), procaine (250 mg) and benethamine (475 mg) penicillins Not resistant to penicillinase Contra-indicated in penicillin-hypersensitivity	IM	1 vial every 2–3 days
Sulphonamides	The main indications for sulphonamides are in the prophylaxis of post-traumatic meningitis but meningococci increasingly are resistant. Co-trimoxazole may be used to treat sinusitis. Contra-indicated in pregnancy and in renal disease. In other patients, adequate hydration must be ensured to prevent the (rare) occurrence of crystalluria. Other adverse reactions include erythema multiforme, rashes and blood dyscrasias		See Section 8.2
Co-trimoxazole	Combination of trimethoprim and sulphamethoxazole Orally active Broad spectrum Occasional rashes or blood dyscrasias Contra-indicated in pregnancy, liver disease May increase the effect of protein-bound drugs	O or IM	960 mg twice daily or 3–4·5 ml IM twice daily
Other sulphonamides	See Table 8.2		
Tetracyclines	Tetracyclines have a broad antibacterial spectrum, but of the many preparations there is little to choose between them. However, doxycycline is useful since a single daily dose is adequate, while minocycline is effective against		

Table 5.8 Some antibacterials (see also Tables 5.22–5.24)—*contd*

	Comments	Route	Dose
	meningococci; both are safer for patients with renal failure. Most other tetracyclines are nephrotoxic. Tetracyclines cause discoloration of developing teeth and have absorption impaired by iron, antacids, milk, etc. Use of tetracyclines may predispose to candidosis, and to nausea and gastrointestinal disturbance		
Tetracycline	Orally active Broad spectrum Contra-indicated in pregnancy and children up to at least 7 years (tooth discoloration) Reduced dose indicated in renal failure, liver disease, elderly Frequent mild gastrointestinal effects	O	250–500 mg 6-hourly
Doxycycline	Orally active Single daily dose Broad spectrum Contra-indicated in pregnancy and children up to at least 7 years (tooth discoloration) Safer than tetracyclines in renal failure (excreted in faeces) Reduce dose in liver disease and elderly Mild gastrointestinal effects	O	100 mg once daily
Minocycline	Orally active Broad spectrum: active against meningococci Safer than tetracycline in renal disease (excreted in faeces) May cause dizziness and vertigo Absorption not reduced by milk Contra-indicated in pregnancy and children up to at least 7 years (tooth discoloration). May rarely also cause tooth or oral pigmentation in adults	O	100 mg twice daily
Vancomycin	Reserved for serious infections, prophylaxis of endocarditis, and treatment of pseudomembranous colitis. Extravenous extravasation causes necrosis and phlebitis May cause nausea, rashes, tinnitus, deafness Rapid injection may cause 'red neck' syndrome Contra-indicated in renal disease, deafness *Very* expensive	O *or* IV	500 mg 6-hourly for pseudomembranous colitis. 1 g IV by slow injection for prophylaxis of endocarditis

Table 5.9 Other antibacterial agents sometimes used in dentistry (see also Tables 5.22–5.24)

	Comments	Route	Dose
Cephalosporins and cephamycins	Cephalosporins are broad spectrum expensive and bactericidal antibiotics with few absolute indications for their use in dentistry, although they may be effective against *Staph. aureus*. They produce false positive results for glucosuria with 'Clinitest'. Hypersensitivity is the main side-effect. Some cause a bleeding tendency. Some are nephrotoxic. Cefuroxime is less affected by penicillinases than other cephalosporins and is currently the preferred drug of the many available		
Cefotaxime and ceftazidime	Not orally active. Broad spectrum activity. Contra-indicated if history of anaphylaxis to penicillin. Expensive	IM or IV	1 g 12-hourly
Cefuroxime	Not orally active. Broad spectrum activity. Contra-indicated if history of anaphylaxis to penicillin	IM or IV	250–750 mg 8-hourly
Cephalexin and cephradine	Orally active Cheaper than most cephalosporins Contra-indicated if history of anaphylaxis to penicillin	O	250–500 mg 6-hourly
Erythromycin	Erythromycin has a similar antibacterial spectrum to penicillin and is therefore used in penicillin-allergic patients. Active against most staphylococci, *Mycoplasma* and *Legionella*, but not always against oral bacteroides. Do not use erythromycin estolate, which may cause liver disease		
Erythromycin stearate	Orally active Useful in those hypersensitive to penicillin Effective against most staphylococci and streptococci. May cause nausea Rapid development of resistance Reduced dose indicated in liver disease. Can increase cyclosporin absorption and toxicity	O	250–500 mg 6-hourly

Table 5.9   Other antibacterial agents sometimes used in dentistry (see also Tables 5.22–5.24)—*contd*

	Comments	Route	Dose
Erythromycin lactobionate	Used where parenteral erythromycin indicated Give not as bolus but by infusion. Comments as above.	IV	2 g daily
Gentamicin	Reserved for use in serious infections and prophylaxis of endocarditis. Can cause vestibular and renal damage especially if given with frusemide Contra-indicated in pregnancy and myasthenia gravis. Reduce dose in renal disease	IM or IV	Up to 5 mg/kg daily
Metronidazole	Orally active Effective against anaerobes Use only for 7 days (or peripheral neuropathy may develop, particularly in liver patients) Avoid alcohol (disulfiram-type reaction) May increase warfarin effect May cause tiredness IV preparation available but expensive. Suppositories are effective Contra-indicated in pregnancy	O or IV	200–400 mg 8-hourly (take with meals)
Rifampicin	Reserved mainly for treatment of tuberculosis. May be used in prophylaxis of meningitis after head injury since *Neisseria meningitidis* may be resistant to sulphonamides. Safe and effective but resistance rapidly occurs. Body secretions turn red. May interfere with oral contraception. Occasional rashes, jaundice or blood dyscrasias		See Section 8.2

Failure of an infection to respond to an antimicrobial within 48 hours should prompt reconsideration of:

- Adequacy of drainage of pus.
- Appropriateness of the antimicrobial and dose.
- Antimicrobial sensitivities of microorganism (staphylococci are now frequently resistant to penicillin and some show multiple resistances—MRSA—multiple resistant *Staphylococcus aureus*).
- Patient compliance.
- Possible local factors (eg foreign body).
- Possibility of unusual type of infection.
- Possibility of impaired host defences (unusual and opportunistic infections are increasingly identified, particularly in the immunocompromised patient).
- Possibility that you are dealing with a non-infective condition!

In serious or unusual cases of infection, consult the clinical microbiologist.

Route of administration

Oral preparations of antimicrobials should be used in most instances. Topical antimicrobials should be avoided, since they may produce sensitisation and may cause the emergence of resistant strains of microorganisms. Parenteral administration of antimicrobials may be indicated where:

- High blood levels are required rapidly (eg serious infections).
- The patient cannot or will not take oral medications (eg unconscious patient).
- The patient is to have a general anaesthetic within the following 4 hours.
- No oral preparation is available (eg vancomycin).

Antifungals

For a list of the more commonly used antifungal agents, see Table 5.10.

Antivirals

At present there are few antiviral agents of proven efficacy. Management of viral infections is therefore predominantly supportive (Table 5.3). Most antivirals will achieve maximum benefit if given early in the disease. Immunocompromised patients with viral infections may well benefit from active antiviral therapy, since these infections may spread locally and systemically (See Table 5.11.).

Table 5.10 Antifungals

	Comments	Oral dose
Amphotericin[a]	Active topically Negligible absorption from gastro-intestinal tract	10–100 mg 6-hourly
Nystatin[a]	Active topically Negligible absorption from gastro-intestinal tract Pastille tastes better than lozenge	500 000 unit lozenge, 100 000 unit pastille or 100 000 unit per ml of suspension 6-hourly
Miconazole[a]	Active topically Also has antibacterial activity Negligible absorption from gastro-intestinal tract Theoretically the best antifungal to treat angular cheilitis	250 mg tablet 6-hourly or 25 mg/ml gel used as 5 ml 6-hourly
Ketoconazole	Absorbed from gastrointestinal tract. Useful in intractable candidosis Contra-indicated in pregnancy and liver disease May cause nausea, rashes, pruritus and liver damage. Enhances nephrotoxicity of cyclosporin	200–400 mg once daily with meal

[a]Dissolve in mouth slowly.

Table 5.11 Antiviral therapy of oral viral infections

Virus	Disease	Otherwise healthy patient	Immunocompromised patient
Herpes simplex	Primary herpetic gingivostomatitis Recurrent herpetic infection, eg herpes labialis	Consider oral acyclovir[ab] 100–200 mg, five times daily as suspension (200 mg/5 ml) or tablets. 5% acyclovir cream	Acyclovir 250 mg/m^2 IV[b] every 8 hours Consider systemic acyclovir[b] as above, depending on risk to patient of infection
Herpes varicella zoster	Chickenpox	—	Acyclovir[b] 500 mg/m^2 (5 mg/kg) IV every 8 hours
	Zoster (shingles)	3% acyclovir ophthalmic ointment for shingles of ophthalmic division of trigeminal	As above

[a]In neonate—treat as if immunocompromised.
[b]Acyclovir: systemic preparations, caution in renal disease and pregnancy, occasional increase in liver enzymes and urea, rashes.

Table 5.12 Examples of topical corticosteroids used in dentistry

Steroid	Dose 6-hourly	Comments
Hydrocortisone hemisuccinate pellets	2·5 mg	Dissolve in mouth close to ulcers; use at an early stage
Triamcinolone acetonide in carmellose gelatin paste	Apply	Adheres best to dry mucosa; affords mechanical protection; of little value on tongue or palate
Betamethasone phosphate tablets	0·5 mg as mouthwash	More potent than preparations above; may produce adrenal suppression
Betamethasone valerate (inhaler)	Spray on lesion 100 μg	More potent than preparations above; may produce adrenal suppression

5.8 Corticosteroids and other immunosuppressive agents

● Topical corticosteroids are useful in the management of many oral ulcers, particularly in recurrent aphthous stomatitis and lichen planus (Table 5.12).

● Intralesional corticosteroids are occasionally useful, for example in the management of intractable erosive lichen planus and keloid scars (see Tables 5.13–5.15).

● Intra-articular corticosteroids are occasionally indicated, for example where there is intractable pain associated with a non-infective arthropathy.

● Systemic corticosteroids are indicated in the management of anaphylaxis (Section 4.10), an adrenal crisis (Section 4.8) and pemphigus. They may also be of value in other disorders, such as giant cell arteritis, Bell's palsy, and can also be used to reduce post-operative or post-traumatic oedema. Because of their serious side-effects (Section 3.4), systemic steroids must always be used with caution. Patients should be given a steroid card and warned of possible adverse reactions.

● Azathioprine may be indicated where prolonged immunosuppression is required, as it has a 'steroid-sparing' effect (Table 5.15).

5.9 Hypnotics (see also Tables 5.16 and 5.17 and Chapters 6 and 7)

● Pain, anxiety or depression may cause insomnia.

● In hospital, patients may temporarily need a hypnotic, but they should not be prescribed without forethought.

Table 5.13   Intralesional corticosteroids

Corticosteroid	Comments	Dose
Prednisolone sodium phosphate	Short-acting	Up to 24 mg
Methylprednisolone acetate	Also available with lignocaine	4–80 mg every 1 to 5 weeks
Triamcinolone acetonide	—	2–3 mg every 1 to 2 weeks
Triamcinolone hexacetonide	—	Up to 5 mg every 3 to 4 weeks

Table 5.14   Intra-articular corticosteroids[a]

Corticosteroid	Comments	Dose
Dexamethasone sodium phosphate	More expensive than hydrocortisone acetate	0·4–5 mg at intervals of 3 to 21 days
Hydrocortisone acetate	Usual preparation used	5–50 mg

[a]Also used are those listed under intralesional corticosteroids

● Hypnotics may be contra-indicated in the elderly and those with liver or respiratory disease. They often potentiate alcohol and other CNS depressants, and they may impair judgement and dexterity.

● Barbiturates and glutethimide should not be used; both are dangerous in overdose, and barbiturates are addictive.

● Benzodiazepines are, in general, the preferred hypnotics, but are contra-indicated in severe respiratory disorders and are also addictive.

5.10 Anxiolytics, sedatives and tranquillisers
General principles

● Identify and treat the cause of the patient's anxiety wherever possible.

● It is important to differentiate between agitated depression and simple anxiety; the treatment is different.

● Doses should be reduced for the elderly, since side-effects, particularly sedation, are common. Beta blockers (eg propranolol) may be more useful if anxiety is causing tremor/palpitations.

● Drowsiness (particularly when used together with alcohol) and impaired judgement are common in patients taking anxiolytics, sedatives or tranquillisers. Patients should therefore be warned of the dangers of driving, operating machinery, or making important decisions.

Table 5.15 Systemic corticosteroids[a] and azathioprine

	Comments	Dose
Prednisolone	In dentistry may be indicated systemically for treatment of pemphigus and Bell's palsy, and occasionally in other disorders (Section 5.8)	Initially 40–80 mg orally each day in divided doses, reducing as soon as possible to 10 mg daily. Give as enteric-coated prednisolone with meals.
Dexamethasone	May be useful to reduce post-surgical oedema after minor surgery	5 mg IV with premedication; then 0·5–1·0 mg each day for 5 days, orally if possible
Betamethasone	May be useful to reduce post-surgical oedema after minor surgery	1 mg orally the night before operation. 1 mg orally with premed. 1 mg IV at operation. 1 mg orally every 6 hours for 2 days post-operatively
Methylprednisolone	May be useful to reduce post-surgical oedema after major surgery	Methylprednisolone sodium succinate 1 g IV at operation then 500 mg IV on the evening of operation, followed by 125 mg IV every 6 hours for 24 hours. Then methylprednisolone acetate 80 mg every 12 hours for 24 hours
Azathioprine[b]	Steroid-sparing for immunosuppression	Orally 2–2·5 mg/kg daily

[a]For details of steroid cover and for treatment of anaphylaxis, see Sections 4.8 and 4.10. See Section 3.4 for serious adverse reactions
[b]Myelosuppressive and hepatotoxic and long-term may predispose to neoplasms. Contra-indicated in pregnancy

- Numerous benzodiazepines are now available. All may produce a degree of dependence (especially lorazepam) and there is often little to choose in terms of anxiolytic effect between the different drugs. Most cause unsteadiness and some confusion.
- Phenothiazines are major tranquillisers and can cause extrapyramidal disorders, postural hypotension, confusion and hypothermia. Chlorpromazine should be avoided in the elderly.
- These drugs should not be stopped suddenly after prolonged or high dosages have been used, as this may precipitate withdrawal symptoms or acute psychosis.

Table 5.16 Hypnotics

Hypnotic	Comments	Preparation contains	Route	Dose (at night)
Chlormethiazole	Contra-indicated in liver disease; useful in elderly; may cause dependence	192 mg capsule or 250 mg/5 ml syrup	O	500 mg
Diazepam	Useful hypnotic; May cause dependence; Reduce dose in elderly;	5 mg or 10 mg	O	5–10 mg
Dichloralphenazone	Derivative of chloral hydrate; contra-indicated in oral anticoagulants, porphyria Useful in elderly	650 mg	O	1300 mg
Nitrazepam	No more useful than diazepam; avoid in elderly; may cause dependence; hangover effect	5 mg	O	5 mg–10 mg
Temazepam	Less 'hangover' effect than nitrazepam; may cause dependence; useful in elderly	10 mg	O	10–20 mg

Table 5.17 Sedatives and tranquillisers (see Table 6.3 for premedication)

	Comments	Preparation contains	Route	Dose
Chlorpromazine	Major tranquilliser May cause dyskinesia, photosensitivity, eye defects and jaundice Contra-indicated in epilepsy. IM use causes pain and may cause postural hypotension	25 mg tab; 25 mg/5 ml syrup; 50 mg/2 ml injection	O *or* IM	25 mg 8-hourly
Chlordiazepoxide	Anxiolytic; reduce dose in elderly	5 mg or 10 mg	O	5–10 mg 8-hourly
Diazepam	Anxiolytic; reduce dose in elderly	2 mg, 5 mg or 10 mg	O	2–30 mg a day in divided doses
Thioridazine	Phenothiazine with fewer adverse effects than chlorpromazine. Major tranquilliser. Rare retinopathy	10 mg or 25 mg	O	10–50 mg 8-hourly
Propranolol	Useful anxiolytic which does not cause amnesia, but reduces tremor and palpitations; contra-indicated in asthma, cardiac failure, pregnancy	10 mg or 40 mg	O	80–100 mg daily
Haloperidol	Major tranquilliser; useful in the elderly; may cause dyskinesia	500 µg	O	500 µg 12-hourly

5.11 Antifibrinolytic agents

Table 5.18 Antifibrinolytic drugs (see also Tables 5.22–5.24)

	Comments	Route	Dose
Epsilon amino caproic acid	Useful in some bleeding tendencies. May cause nausea, diarrhoea, dizziness, myalgia. Contra-indicated in pregnancy: history of thromboembolism; renal disease	O	3 g, 4–6 times daily
Tranexamic acid	Comments as above, but tranexamic acid is usually the preferred drug	O	1–1·5 g, 6- or 12-hourly
		IV	Slow IV injection 1 g, 8-hourly

5.12 Hepatitis vaccines

Table 5.19   Immunisation against hepatitis B

Vaccine	Comments	Dose
Hepatitis B vaccine	Useful in individuals at high risk of contracting viral hepatitis B and HB_sAb neg.	3 doses each of 1 ml. Second dose 1 month, third 6 months after initial dose[a]
Anti-hepatitis B virus immunoglobulin	Contact consultant microbiologist or Public Health Laboratory Service	

[a] Booster needed every 3–5 years.

5.13 Other drugs

Table 5.20   Other drugs (see also Tables 5.22–5.24)

Drug	Comments	Route	Dose
Etretinate	Vitamin A analogue may be used in treatment of erosive lichen planus. Effect begins after 2 to 3 weeks. Treat for 6 to 9 months, followed by a similar rest period. Most patients develop dry, cracked lips. May cause epistaxis, pruritus, alopecia. Contra-indicated in pregnancy: liver disease.	O	0·5–1 mg/kg daily in two divided doses
Carbamazepine	Prophylactic for trigeminal neuralgia—not analgesic. Occasional dizziness, diplopia, and blood dyscrasia, usually with a rash and usually in the first 3 months of treatment. Potentiated by cimetidine, dextropropoxyphene and isoniazid. Potentiates lithium.	O	Initially 100 mg once or twice daily. Many patients need about 200 mg 8-hourly. Do not exceed 1800 mg daily.

5.14 Adverse reactions to drugs

Almost any drug may produce unwanted or unexpected adverse reactions; never use any drug unless there are good indications (see Tables 5.21–5.24.) The true incidence of adverse drug reactions is often not known, and many adverse reactions are probably not, at present, recognised as drug-related. Always take a full medical history and ask specifically about adverse drug reactions, since the medical status may influence the choice of drugs used.

Avoid polypharmacy, and use only drugs with which you are familiar.

Drugs can cause a wide range of adverse reactions affecting the mouth (Table 5.21). Patients should be warned if serious adverse reactions are liable to occur (eg systemic corticosteroids), and provided with the appropriate warning card to carry.

The only way to improve recognition of adverse drug reactions is to record any possible reactions, which, in the UK, should be reported (on the yellow prepaid postcards available from the Committee on Safety of Medicines) to:

> The Medical Assessor (Adverse Reactions)
> The Committee on Safety of Medicines and
>   Dental and Surgical Materials
> Market Towers
> 1 Nine Elms Lane
> London SW8 5BR
> (Tel: 01-720 2188)

5.15 Drug information services

Information on any aspect of drug therapy can be obtained, free of charge, from Regional and District Drug Information Services. Details regarding the *local* services provided within your Region can be obtained by telephoning the following numbers.

England

Birmingham	021-378 2211	Extn 3565
Bristol	0272 260256	Direct Line
Guildford	0483 504312	Direct line
Ipswich	0473 712233	Extn 4322/4323
	or 0473 718687	Direct Line
Leeds	0532 430715	Direct Line
Leicester	0533 555779	Direct Line
Liverpool	051-236 4620	Extn 2126/2127/2128
London (Guy's Hospital)	01-407 7600	Extn 2548
London (London Hospital)	01-377 7487	Direct Line
	or 01-377 7488	Direct Line
London (Northwick Park)	01-423 4535	Direct Line
Manchester	061-225 2063	Direct Line
	or 061-276 6270	Direct Line
Newcastle	091-232 1525	Direct Line
Oxford	0865 742424	Direct Line
Southampton	0703 780323	Direct Line

Northern Ireland
  Belfast   0232 248095   Direct Line
  Londonderry   0504 45171   Extn 3262

Scotland
  Aberdeen   0224 681818   Extn 52316
  Dundee   0382 60111   Extn 2351
  Edinburgh   031-229 2477 Extn 2234/2936
  Glasgow   041-552 4726 Direct Line
  Inverness   0463 234151   Extn 288
                              or 0463 220157   Direct Line

Wales
  Cardiff   0222 759541   Direct Line

Poisons Information Services

Belfast   0232 240503
Birmingham   021-554 3801
Cardiff   0222 709901
Dublin   0001 379964
               or 0001 379966
Edinburgh   031-229 2477
               031-228 2441
               (Viewdata)
Leeds   0532 430715
               or 0532 432799
London   01-635 9191
               or 01-407 7600
Newcastle   091-232 5131

Table 5.21 Oral side-effects of drug treatment (most are rare, but the more common causes are printed in italic)

Tooth discoloration
Chlorhexidine
Fluorides
Iron
Tetracyclines[a]

Oral candidosis
Broad-spectrum antimicrobials
Corticosteroids
Drugs causing xerostomia
Immunosuppressives

Oral ulceration
Cocaine
Cytotoxics
Emepromium
Gold
Indomethacin
Isoprenaline
Naproxen
Pancreatin
Penicillamine
Phenindione
Phenytoin
Phenylbutazone
Potassium chloride
Proguanil

Facial pain
Phenothiazines
Stilbamidine
Vinca alkaloids

Erythema multiforme
(and Stevens Johnson syndrome)
Barbiturates
Busulphan
Carbamazepine
Clindamycin
Codeine
Frusemide
Penicillin
Phenylbutazone
Phenytoin
Sulphonamides
Tetracyclines

Angioedema
Aspirin

Essential oils
Penicillin

Gingival hyperplasia
Contraceptive pill
Cyclosporin
Diltiazem
Nifedipine
Phenytoin

Oral mucosal pigmentation
ACTH
Amodiaquine
Anticonvulsants
Busulphan
Chlorhexidine
Chloroquine
Contraceptive pill
Heavy metals
Mepacrine
Minocycline
Phenothiazines
Smoking

Lichenoid reactions
Amiphenazole
Chloroquine
Chlorpropamide
Dapsone
Gold
Labetalol
Mepacrine
Methyldopa
Non steroidal anti-inflammatory drugs (NSAIDS)
Oxprenolol
Para-aminosalicylate
Penicillamine
Phenothiazines
Practolol
Propranolol
Quinine
Quinidine
Streptomycin
Tetracycline
Thiazides
Tolbutamide
Triprolidine

Lupoid reactions
Ethosuximide
Gold
Griseofulvin
Hydralazine
Isoniazid
Methyldopa
Para-aminosalicylate
Penicillin
Phenytoin
Procainamide
Streptomycin
Sulphonamides
Tetracyclines

Pemphigus-like reactions
Captopril
Penicillamine
Rifampicin

Pemphigoid-like reactions
Clonidine
Frusemide
Penicillamine
Psoralens

Salivary gland swelling
Anti-thyroid agents
Chlorhexidine
Cimetidine
Clonidine
Ganglion-blocking agents
Insulin
Interferon
Iodides
Isoprenaline
Methyldopa
Nitrofurantoin
Oxyphenbutazone
Phenothiazines
Phenylbutazone
Sulphonamides

Salivary gland pain
Bethanidine
Clonidine
Cytotoxics
Guanethidine
Methyldopa

Table 5.21   Oral side-effects of drug treatment (most are rare, but the more common causes are printed in italic)—*contd*

Hypersalivation	Captopril	Tetrabenazine
Anticholinesterases	Carbimazole	Tricyclics
Buprenorphine	Clofibrate	
Ethionamide	Dipyridamole	**Trigeminal paraesthesia**
Iodides	Ethionamide	*Acetazolamide*
Ketamine	Gold	Ergotamine
Mercurials	Griseofulvin	Hydralazine
Niridazole	Guanoclor	Isoniazid
	Lincomycin	*Labetalol*
Xerostomia	Lithium	Methysergide
Amphetamines	Metformin	Monoamine oxidase
Antihistamines	*Metronidazole*	inhibitors
Atropinics	Niridazole	Nalidixic acid
Benzhexol	Penicillamine	Nitrofurantoin
Benztropine	Phenindione	Phenytoin
Biperiden	Prothionamide	Propofol
Clonidine		Propranolol
L-dopa	**Cervical lymph node**	Stilbamidine
Ganglion-blocking agents	**enlargement**	Streptomycin
Lithium	Phenytoin	Sulphonylureas
Monoamine oxidase	Phenylbutazone	*Sulthiame*
inhibitors	Primidone	Tricyclics
Opiates		
Orphenadrine	**Involuntary facial**	**Labial crusting**
Phenothiazines	**movements**	Etretinate
Propantheline	Butyrophenones	
Selegiline	Carbamazepine	**Scalded mouth sensation**
Tricyclics	L-dopa	Captopril
	Lithium	
	Methyldopa	**Halitosis**
Disturbed taste	Metoclopramide	Disulfiram
Anti-thyroids	*Phenothiazines*	DMSO
Biguanides	Phenytoin	Isorbide dinitrate

[a] Minocycline can cause tooth staining in *adults*; any tetracycline can discolour developing teeth.

See Tables 5.22–5.24 for further information on drugs and their contra-indications.

Diseases and abnormalities
of the oral tissues

The following section consists of illustrations of a number of conditions which may be seen in the oral cavity, and which the dentist should be able to diagnose and treat, as appropriate. All these are mentioned in the text, but are not cross-referenced to this section.

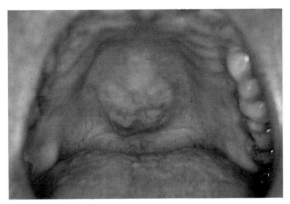

Torus palatinus.

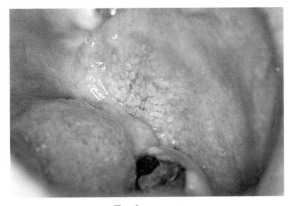

Fordyce spots.

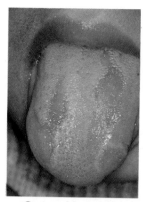

Geographic tongue.

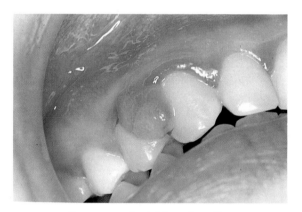

Pregnancy gingivitis and epulis.

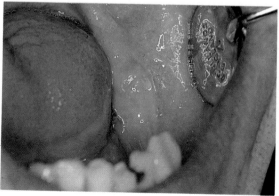

Odontogenic cyst.

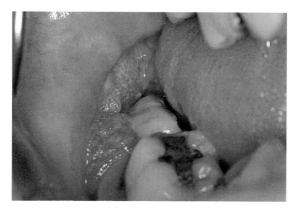

Squamous carcinoma.

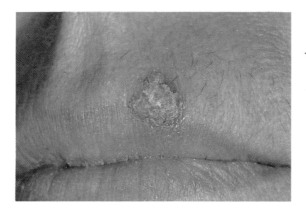

Recurrent herpes labialis.

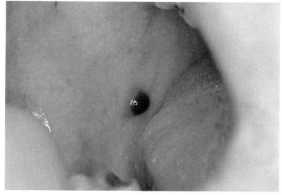

Blood blister, in this instance due to localised oral purpura.

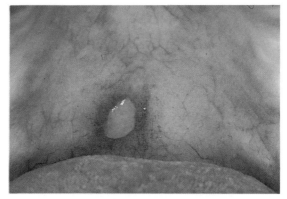

Bulla, in mucous membrane pemphigoid.

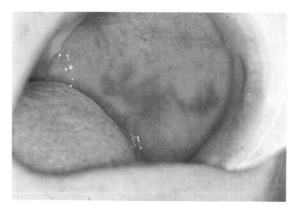

A rare case of pigmentation caused by Addison's disease.

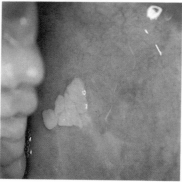

Keratosis (homogenous leukoplakia).

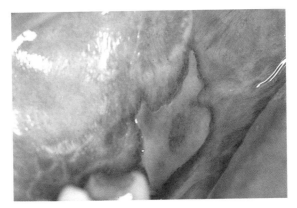

Lichen planus (erosive type).

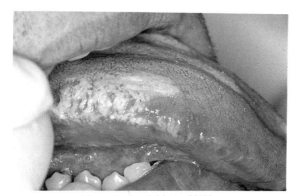

Hairy leukoplakia in HIV.

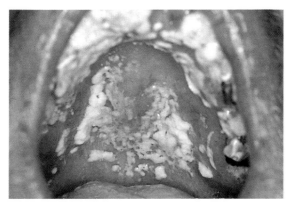

This case of thrush is highly suggestive of HIV.

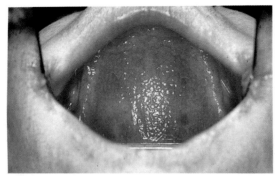

Denture-induced stomatitis.

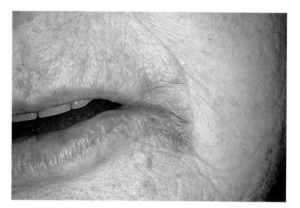

Angular stomatitis.

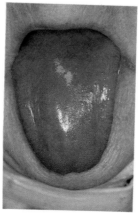

Lingual depapillation.

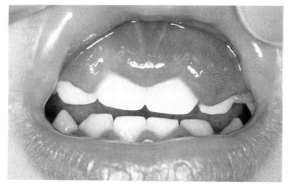

Herpetic stomatitis.

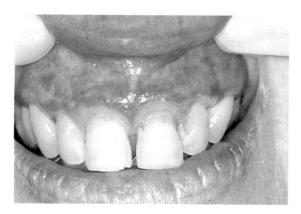

Desquamative gingivitis.

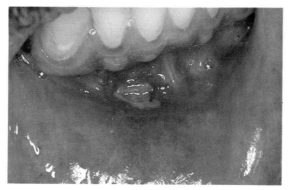

Aphthous ulcer.

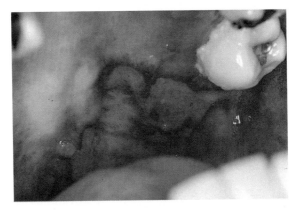

Pemphigoid.

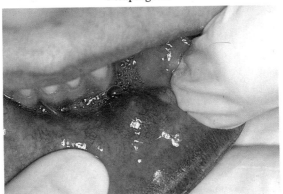

Mucocele.

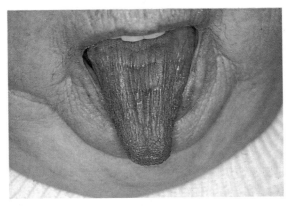

Xerostomia.

Table 5.22 Drugs to be avoided or used only in reduced doses for specific conditions

Condition	Drug that may be contra-indicated[a]	Condition	Drug that may be contra-indicated[a]
Addison's disease (hypoadreno-corticism)	Any general anaesthetic Methohexitone Thiopentone	Elderly	Atropinics Diazepam[b] Dihydrocodeine Ketamine NSAIDS Tricyclics
Alcoholism	Aspirin Metronidazole Any general anaesthetic	Epilepsy	Enflurane Flumazenil Ketamine Methohexitone Phenothiazines Tricyclics
Allergies	Aspirin Methohexitone Penicillin		
Asthma	Aspirin NSAIDS Opiates	Glaucoma	Atropinics Carbamazepine Diazepam[b]
Bleeding disorders	Aspirin Corticosteroids	Glucose-6-phosphate dehydrogenase deficiency	Aspirin Co-trimoxazole Sulphonamides
Burns	Suxamethonium		
Carcinoid syndrome	Opiates	Gout	Aspirin Amoxycillin Ampicillin
Cardiovascular diseases	Adrenaline Chloral hydrate Halothane Methohexitone Pentazocine Propanidid Thiopentone Tricyclics	Head injury	Ketamine Opiates
		Hypertension	Adrenaline Corticosteroids Ketamine Pentazocine
Cerebrovascular disease	Diazepam[b]	Hyperthyroidism	Adrenaline Atropinics
Chronic lymphocytic leukaemia	Amoxycillin Ampicillin	Hypothyroidism	Any general anaesthetic Codeine Diazepam[b] Dihydrocodeine Methohexitone Opiates Pethidine Thiopentone
Children under 7 years	Aspirin Tetracyclines		
Constipation	Codeine		
Diabetes mellitus	Aspirin Corticosteroids		
Diarrhoea	Mefenamic acid Clindamycin	Infectious mononucleosis	Amoxycillin Ampicillin
Drug addiction	Pentazocine	Liver disease (See also Table 3.19)	Any general anaesthetic Antidepressants
Dystrophia myo-tonica (myotonic dystrophy)	Methohexitone Suxamethonium Thiopentone		

Table 5.22   Drugs to be avoided or used only in reduced doses for specific conditions—*contd*

Condition	Drug that may be contra-indicated[a]	Condition	Drug that may be contra-indicated[a]
	Aspirin		Metronidazole
	Carbamazepine		MAOI
	Carbenoxolone		Sulphonamides
	Chloral hydrate		Thiopentone
	Clindamycin	Pregnancy[c]	Care with all drugs
	Corticosteroids	(See also Table 3.22)	Aspirin
	Co-trimoxazole		Co-trimoxazole
	Dextro-propoxyphene		Diazepam[b]
	Diazepam[b]		Epsilon amino
	Erythromycin		caproic acid
	estolate		Etretinate
	Etretinate		Flumazenil
	Flumazenil		Mefenamic acid
	Halothane		Opiates
	Ketoconazole		Sulphonamides
	Methohexitone		Tetracyclines
	Opiates or codeine	Parkinsonism	Benzodiazepines
	Paracetamol		
	Pentazocine	Psychiatric disease	Ketamine
	Phenothiazines	Raised intracranial	Ketamine
	Rifampicin	pressure	Opiates
	Suxamethonium		
	Thiopentone	Renal disease	Any general
	Tricyclics	(See also Table 3.2)	anaesthetic or
Malignant	Halothane		CNS depressant
hyperpyrexia	Ketamine		or NSAID
	Suxamethonium		Acyclovir (systemic)
			Aspirin
Neuromuscular	Diazepam[b]		Carbamazepine
diseases	Methohexitone		Cephaloridine
	Suxamethonium		Cephalothin
	Tetracyclines		Chloral hydrate
	Thiopentone		Clindamycin
			Co-trimoxazole
Peptic ulcer	Aspirin		Diazepam[b]
	Chloral hydrate		Dihydrocodeine
	Corticosteroids		Mefenamic acid
	Mefenamic acid		Metronidazole
			Opiates
Phaeochromo-	Adrenaline		Paracetamol
cytoma	Barbiturates		Sulphonamides
	Enflurane		Suxamethonium
			Tetracyclines
Porphyria	Co-trimoxazole	Respiratory disease	Any general
	Carbamazepine		anaesthetic
	Dextropro-		Dextro-
	poxyphene		propoxyphene
	Diazepam[b]		Diazepam[b]
	Erythromycin		
	Methohexitone		

Table 5.22 Drugs to be avoided or used only in reduced doses for specific conditions—*contd*

Condition	Drug that may be contra-indicated[a]	Condition	Drug that may be contra-indicated[a]
Respiratory disease (*contd*)	Dihydrocodeine Methohexitone Opiates Thiopentone	Teenagers	Metoclopramide
		Thrombotic disease	Epsilon amino caproic acid Tranexamic acid
Suxamethonium sensitivity	Suxamethonium	Tuberculosis	Corticosteroids
Systemic lupus erythematosus	Tetracyclines	Urinary retention (prostatic disease)	Atropinics Opiates

[a] Contra-indications are often relative, or of theoretical interest only; other drugs may also be contra-indicated.

[b] Midazolam *may* be safer but should still be used with caution.

[c] And breast-feeding.

Table 5.23   Disease contra-indications to drugs used in dentistry

Drug	Possible contra-indications	Possible reaction
Acyclovir (systemic)	Renal disease	Urea rises
Adrenaline	Hypertension	Hypertension
	Hyperthyroidism	Arrhythmias
	Ischaemic heart disease	Arrhythmias
	Phaeochromocytoma	Hypertension
Ampicillin	Allergy to penicillin	Anaphylaxis
(or amoxycillin)	Chronic lymphocytic leukaemia	Rash
or derivatives	Gout	Rash
	Infectious mononucleosis	Rash
Aspirin	Allergy to aspirin including aspirin-induced asthma	Anaphylaxis
	Alcoholism	Gastric bleeding
	Bleeding disorders	Gastric bleeding
	Breast-feeding	Reye's syndrome
	Children	Reye's syndrome
	Diabetes	Interferes with control
	Glucose 6-phosphate-dehydrogenase	Haemolysis
	Gout	Gout worse
	Liver disease	Bleeding tendency
	Peptic ulcer	Gastric bleeding
	Pregnancy	Haemorrhage
	Renal disease	Fluid retention and gastric bleeding
Atropinics	Glaucoma	Raised intra-ocular pressure
	Hyperthyroidism	Tachycardias
	The elderly	Confusion: urine retention
	Urinary retention or prostatic hypertrophy	Urinary retention
Carbamazepine	Glaucoma	Raised intra-ocular pressure
	Liver disease	Hepatotoxic
	Porphyria	Acute porphyria
	The elderly	Agitation or confusion
Carbenoxolone	Liver disease	Toxicity
Cephalosporins[a]	Allergy to cephalosporins	Anaphylaxis
	Allergy to penicillins	Allergy
	Renal disease	Nephrotoxic
Chloral hydrate	Cardiovascular disease	Fluid retention
	Gastritis	Gastric irritation
	Liver disease	Coma
	Renal disease	CNS depression
Clindamycin	Liver disease	Increased toxicity
	Renal disease	Increased toxicity
Codeine	Colonic disease	Constipation
	Liver disease	Respiratory depression
	Hypothyroidism	Coma

Table 5.23 Disease contra-indications to drugs used in dentistry—*contd*

Drug	Possible contra-indications	Possible reaction
Corticosteroids	Diabetes mellitus	Diabetes worsened
	Hypertension	Increased hypertension
	Peptic ulcer	Perforation
	Tuberculosis	Possible dissemination
Co-trimoxazole	Elderly	Agranulocytosis
	Glucose-6-phosphate-dehydrogenase deficiency	Haemolysis
	Liver disease	Enhanced toxicity
	Porphyria	Acute porphyria
	Pregnancy	Folate deficiency
	Renal disease	Increased toxicity
Dextro-propoxyphene	Liver disease	Potentiated
	Respiratory disease	Respiratory depression
	Pregnancy	Foetal depression
Diazepam	Cerebrovascular disease	Cerebral ischaemia
	Chronic obstructive airways disease	Respiratory depression
	Glaucoma	Increased ocular pressure
	Hypothyroidism	Coma
	Neuromuscular disorders	Condition deteriorates
	Porphyria	Acute porphyria
	Pregnancy	Foetal hypoxia
	Severe kidney disease	Increased diazepam effect
	Severe liver disease	Increased diazepam effect
	Elderly	Cerebral ischaemia
Dihydrocodeine	Hypothyroidism	Coma
	Renal disease	Increased toxicity
	Respiratory disease	Respiratory depression
	The elderly	Increased toxicity
Enflurane	Epilepsy	Epileptogenic
Epsilon amino caproic acid	Haematuria	Renal tract obstruction
	Pregnancy	Thrombosis
	Thrombotic disease	Thrombosis
Erythromycin estolate	Liver disease	Hepatotoxic
Etretinate	Liver disease	Hepatotoxic
	Pregnancy	Teratogenic
Flumazenil	Allergy	Allergy
	Epilepsy	Epileptogenic
	Liver disease	Delayed excretion
	Pregnancy	Teratogenic
Halothane	Cardiac arrhythmias	Increased arrhythmias
	Halothane hepatitis	Hepatitis
	Malignant hyperpyrexia	Pyrexia
	Recent anaesthesia with halothane	Hepatitis

Table 5.23   Disease contra-indications to drugs used in dentistry—*contd*

Drug	Possible contra-indications	Possible reaction
Ketamine	Adults	Hallucinations
	Epilepsy	Fits
	Hypertension	Hypertension
	Malignant hyperpyrexia	Pyrexia
	Psychiatric disease	Psychotic reactions
	Raised intracranial pressure	Increased intracranial pressure
Ketoconazole	Liver disease	Hepatotoxic
Lincomycin	(*as for* Clindamycin)	
Mefenamic acid	Asthma	Bronchospasm
	Diarrhoea	Diarrhoea worse
	Peptic ulcer	Bleeding
	Pregnancy and lactation	Teratogenic?
	Renal disease	Renal damage
Methohexitone	Addison's disease	Coma
	Allergies	Anaphylaxis
	Barbiturate sensitivity	Anaphylaxis
	Cardiovascular disease	Cardiovascular depression
	Dystrophia myotonica	Increased weakness
	Epilepsy	Epileptogenic
	Hypothyroidism	Coma
	Liver disease	Increased anaesthesia
	Myasthenia gravis	Increased weakness
	Porphyria	Acute porphyria
	Post-nasal drip	Laryngeal spasm
	Respiratory disease	Respiratory depression
Metoclopramide	Teenagers	Dystonic reactions
Metronidazole	Blood dyscrasias	Leucopenia
	CNS disease	Neuropathy
	Porphyria	Acute porphyria
	Renal disease	Increased drug effect
	Pregnancy	Teratogenic?
Midazolam	(*as for* Diazepam)	
NSAIDS	Asthma*	Bronchospasm
	Peptic ulcer	Gastric bleeding
	Pregnancy	Patent ductus arteriosus
	Renal disease	Nephrotoxic
Opiates	Asthma	Bronchospasm
	Carcinoid tumour	Increased toxicity
	Chronic obstructive airways disease	Respiratory depression
	Head injury	Confuse 'eye signs'
	Hypothyroidism	Coma
	Liver disease	Increased respiratory depression
	Pregnancy	Foetal depression
	Renal disease	Increased respiratory depression
	Urinary retention or prostatic enlargement	Urinary retention

Table 5.23 Disease contra-indications to drugs used in dentistry–*contd*

Drug	Possible contra-indications	Possible reaction
Paracetamol	Liver disease	Hepatotoxicity
	Renal disease	Nephrotoxicity
Penicillins	Allergy to penicillin	Anaphylaxis
	Renal disease	Hyperkalaemia with IM benzyl penicillin
Pentazocine	Hypertension	Hypertension
	Liver disease	Enhanced activity
	Myocardial infarct (recent)	Cardiac arrest
	Narcotic addict	Withdrawal syndrome
	Pregnancy	Foetal depression
Pethidine	Hypothyroidism	Coma
Promethazine	Liver disease	Coma
Rifampicin	Liver disease	Hepatotoxic
Sulphonamides	Glucose-6-phosphate dehydrogenase deficiency	Haemolysis
	Porphyria	Acute porphyria
	Pregnancy	Foetal haemolysis
	Renal disease[b]	Crystalluria
Suxamethonium	Burns	Arrhythmias
	Dystrophia myotonica	Increased muscle weakness
	Liver disease	Apnoea
	Malignant hyperpyrexia	Pyrexia
	Myasthenia gravis	Increased muscle weakness
	Renal disease	Apnoea
	Suxamethonium sensitivity	Apnoea
Tetracyclines	After gastrointestinal surgery	Enterocolitis
	Children under 7	Tooth staining
	Myasthenia gravis	Increased muscle weakness
	Pregnancy	Tooth staining (foetus)
	Renal disease[c]	Nephrotoxicity
	Systemic lupus erythematosus	Photosensitivity
Thiopentone	Addison's disease	Coma
	Barbiturate sensitivity	Anaphylaxis
	Cardiovascular disease	Cardiovascular depression
	Dystrophia myotonica	Increased weakness
	Hypothyroidism	Coma
	Liver disease	Increased anaesthesia
	Myasthenia gravis	Increased weakness
	Porphyria	Acute porphyria
	Post-nasal drip	Laryngeal spasm
	Respiratory disease	Respiratory depression
Tranexamic acid	Haematuria frequency	Renal tract obstruction
	Pregnancy	Thromboses
Triclofos	Thromboembolic disease	Thromboses

Table 5.23   Disease contra-indications to drugs used in dentistry—*contd*

Drug	Possible contra-indications	Possible reaction
Tricyclics	(*see* Chloral hydrate)	Postural hypotension: arrhythmias
	Cardiovascular disease	Increased fits
	Epilepsy	Increased drug effect
	Liver disease	Confusion
	The elderly	Hypotension

Note: Many of these reactions are likely to be of more theoretical interest than clinical significance, so that reference should also be made to the appropriate chapters for particular diseases.
[a] Some cephalosporins give a false positive reaction for glycosuria
[b] Not sulphadimidine
[c] Not doxycycline or minocycline

Table 5.24   Possible drug interactions in dentistry

Drug used in dentistry	Drug	Possible effects
Adrenaline	Halothane	Arrhythmias
	Tricyclics	Pressor response in overdose
Anaesthetics (general)	Antihypertensives	Hypotension
	MAOI	Enhanced hypotension; anaesthetics potentiated
Antibiotics	Oral anticoagulants	Enhanced anticoagulant effect
	Oral contraceptive	Reduced contraception
Aspirin	Alcohol	Increased risk of gastric bleeding
	Corticosteroids	Increased liability of peptic ulceration
	Methotrexate	Enhanced methotrexate activity
	Metoclopramide	Potentiation
	Oral anticoagulants	Enhanced anticoagulant effect
	Oral hypoglycaemics	Enhanced hypoglycaemic effect
Phenylbutazone	Increased liability of peptic ulceration	
	Probenecid	Uricosuric action reduced
	Sodium valproate	Bleeding tendency
	Sulphinpyrazone	Uricosuric action reduced
Atropine	Metoclopramide	Antagonism
Barbiturates	Alcohol	May be increased sedation or resistance
	Antihypertensives	Hypotension
	Antihistamines	Enhanced sedation
	Corticosteroids	May precipitate hypotensive crises

Table 5.24 Possible drug interactions in dentistry—*contd*

Drug used in dentistry	Drug	Possible effects
	Cyclosporin	Reduced effect of cyclosporin
	MAOI	Enhanced sedation
	Oral anticoagulants	Reduced anticoagulant activity
	Phenothiazines	Tremor
	Tricyclics	Cardiac arrest
Carbamazepine	Contraceptive pill	Reduced efficacy of 'pill'
	Cyclosporin	Reduced effect of cyclosporin
	Dextropropoxyphene	Enhanced effect of carbamazepine
	Doxycycline	Reduced doxycycline effect
	Erythromycin	Carbamazepine toxicity
	Lithium	Lithium toxicity
	MAOI	Possible hypertension
	Oral anticoagulants	Reduced anticoagulant effect
	Phenytoin	Reduced phenytoin effect
	Sodium valproate	Reduced effect of valproate
Cephalosporins	Oral anticoagulants	Increased bleeding tendency
	Diuretics	Increased nephrotoxicity
Codeine	MAOI	Coma
Corticosteroids	Aspirin or other analgesics	Increased liability of peptic ulceration
	Cyclosporin or other immunosuppressives	Increased immuno- suppressives.
	Oral anticoagulants	Gastric bleeding
Co-trimoxazole	Methotrexate	Possible folate deficiency
	Oral anticoagulants	Increased bleeding
	Oral contraceptive	Reduced contraceptive effect
	Oral hypoglycaemics	Enhanced hypoglycaemia
	Phenytoin	Phenytoin toxicity
Dextropropoxyphene	Alcohol	Central nervous system depression
	Carbamazepine	Enhanced effect of carbamazepine
	Oral anticoagulants	Enhanced anticoagulant effect
	Orphenadrine	Tremor, anxiety and confusion
Diazepam and other sedatives	Antihistamines	Enhanced sedation
	Cimetidine	Enhanced sedation
	Halothane	Enhanced activity of halothane
	L-dopa	Antagonism
	Lithium	Hypothermia
	Pentazocine and opiates	Respiratory depression
	Phenytoin	Phenytoin toxicity
	Suxamethonium	Activity of suxamethonium reduced
	Tricyclics	Enhanced sedation
Ephedrine	MAOI	Hypertension
	Tricyclics	Hypertension

Table 5.24 Possible drug interactions in dentistry—*contd*

Drug used in dentistry	Drug	Possible effects
Erythromycin	Carbamazepine	Carbamazepine toxicity
	Cyclosporin	Increased cyclosporin absorption
	Oral anticoagulants	Increased bleeding
	Theophyllines	Toxicity
Flumazenil	Tricyclics	Sedation
Gentamicin	Frusemide	Toxicity and nephrotoxicity
Halothane	Aminophylline	Arrhythmias
	Anticonvulsants	Phenytoin toxicity
	Antihypertensives	Hypotension
	Diazepam	Enhanced activity of halothane
	Fenfluramine	Arrhythmias
	Isoprenaline	Arrhythmias
	L-dopa	Arrhythmias
	Lithium	Arrhythmias
	Opiates	Respiratory depression
	Phenothiazines	Respiratory depression; hypotension
Ketamine	CNS depressants	Increased sedation
Ketoconazole	Cyclosporin	Nephrotoxicity
Monoamine oxidase inhibitors	Antihypertensives	Reduced *or* increased hypotensive effect
	Codeine	Hypertension
	General anaesthesia	Hypertension
	L-dopa	Hypertensive crisis
	Methohexitone	Hypotension
	Opiates	Respiratory depression
	Oral anticoagulants	Enhanced anticoagulant effect
	Oral hypoglycaemia	Enhanced hypoglycaemia
	Pethidine	Hypertensive crisis
	Propranolol	Hypertensive crisis
	Tricyclics	Excitation and other interactions
	Tyramine-containing foods	Hypertensive crisis
Mefenamic acid	Oral anticoagulants	Enhanced anticoagulant effect
	Oral hypoglycaemics	Enhanced hypoglycaemia
Methohexitone	Alcohol	Increased sedation
	Antihypertensives	Hypotension
	MAOI	Coma
	Opiates incl. pentazocine	Respiratory depression
	Phenothiazines	Respiratory depression or hypotension; tremor
Metronidazole	Alcohol	Headache and hypotension
	Oral anticoagulants	Increased bleeding tendency
Midazolam	(*as for* Diazepam)	

Table 5.24 Possible drug interactions in dentistry—*contd*

Drug used in dentistry	Drug	Possible effects
Noradrenaline	Tricyclics	Hypertension
NSAIDS	Cyclosporin	Nephrotoxicity
	Oral anticoagulants	Increased bleeding tendency
	Lithium	Lithium toxicity
Opiates	Halothane	Respiratory depression
	MAOI	Respiratory depression or coma
	Methohexitone	Respiratory depression
Paracetamol	Cholestyramine	Reduced absorption of paracetamol
	Metoclopramide	Potentiation
	Oral anticoagulants	Increased bleeding tendency
	Zidovudine	Increased myelosuppression
Pentazocine	Diazepam	Respiratory depression
Pethidine	MAOI	Hypertensive crisis
	Phenothiazines	Respiratory depression
Phenothiazines	Alcohol	May be increased sedation
	Antihistamines	Enhanced sedation
	Antihypertensives	Hypotension
	Barbiturates	Tremor
	Oral anticoagulants	Enhanced anticoagulant effect
	Pethidine	Respiratory depression
	Tricyclics	Convulsions
Phenylbutazone	Aspirin	Increased liability of peptic ulceration
Promethazine	Methohexitone	Increased side-effects of methohexitone
Rifampicin	Cyclosporin	Reduced effect of cyclosporin
	Oral contraceptive	Reduced contraceptive effect
	Oral anticoagulant	Reduced bleeding tendency
Sulphonamides	Methotrexate	Increased methotrexate toxicity
	Oral anticoagulants	Enhanced anticoagulant effect
	Oral hypoglycaemics	Enhanced hypoglycaemia
	Phenytoin	Phenytoin toxicity
Suxamethonium	Cytotoxic drugs	Prolonged muscle paralysis
	Diazepam	Activity of suxamethonium reduced
	Diethylstilboestrol	Prolonged muscle paralysis
	Ecothiopate	Prolonged muscle paralysis
	Digitalis	Digitalis toxicity enhanced
	Lithium	Onset of suxamethonium delayed, action prolonged
	Propanidid	Enhanced muscle paralysis
	Spironolactone	Plasma potassium rises; potential arrhythmias

Table 5.24   Possible drug interactions in dentistry—*contd*

Drug used in dentistry	Drug	Possible effects
Tetracyclines	Antacids	Lower serum levels of tetracyclines
	Barbiturates	Reduced doxycycline blood levels
	Cimetidine	Reduced serum tetracycline levels
	Iron	Reduced serum tetracycline levels
	Methoxyflurane	Renal damage
	Milk	Reduced tetracycline absorption
	Oral anticoagulants	Bleeding tendency
	Oral contraceptive	Reduced contraceptive effect
Thiopentone	Alcohol	Increased sedation
	Antihypertensives	Hypotension
	MAOI	Coma
	Opiates	Respiratory depression
	Phenothiazines	Respiratory depression
Tricyclics	Sulphonamides	Barbiturate potentiated
	Adrenaline	Hypertensive response in overdose
	Alcohol	Enhanced central nervous system
	Anaesthetics	(see Barbiturates)
	Antihypertensives	Impaired blood pressure control
	Atropinics	Enhanced atropinic effects
	Diazepam	Enhanced sedation
	MAOI	Excitation and other interactions
	Oral anticoagulants	Enhanced anticoagulant effect
	Phenothiazines	Convulsions

Note: Many of these drug interactions are of little more than theoretical importance in dentistry, or are the result of overdose of one or both agents. However, there can be wide individual variations in response to drugs, especially sedating agents.

6

Local Analgesia, Conscious Sedation and General Anaesthesia

Most dental patients are satisfactorily treated with local analgesia (LA) alone. Certain handicapped individuals, some nervous children and adults undergoing emergency treatment, and any patient undergoing extensive oral surgery will require general anaesthesia (GA). A remaining small group may be best treated using local analgesia together with conscious sedation, but this should never be allowed to take the place of good patient management and satisfactory pain control.

6.1 Choice of technique: possible medical contra-indications to general anaesthesia (Tables 6.1, 6.5)

General anaesthesia may be contra-indicated if the patient has taken anything except plain water by mouth in the previous 4–6 hours.

Table 6.1 Choice of sedation and anaesthesia

Procedure	Indications	Contra-indications
Local analgesia	Analgesia for simple operations or when GA contra-indicated	Uncooperative patient Infected injection site Bleeding disorders Extensive or major procedures
Conscious sedation	Anxious patient Mentally handicapped	Cardiorespiratory, liver, kidney or psychiatric disease[a] Unescorted patient[a] Adverse reaction to agent[a]
General anaesthesia	LA not effective, eg acute abscess Extensive or major procedures Uncooperative patient, eg handicapped Bleeding disorders	Medical disorders,[b] eg respiratory disease Respiratory obstruction Recent meal[c] Unescorted patient Adverse reaction to agent

[a] Contra-indications to IV sedation mainly.
[b] See Section 6.1.
[c] Within the previous 4 hours (longer in the traumatised patient, and in those with head injury 12–24 hours may be needed).

Table 6.2   Local anaesthetic agents[a]

Agent	Comments	Maximum safe dose for fit adults
Lignocaine 2% plain	Poor and brief analgesia (15–45 minutes)	200 mg (5 × 2-ml cartridges)
Lignocaine 2% plus adrenaline[b] 1 in 80 000	Effective analgesia for > 90 minutes	500 mg (12 × 2-ml cartridges)
Prilocaine 4% plain	Poor and brief analgesia (circa 30 minutes) Methaemoglobinaemia in excess	400 mg (6 × 2-ml cartridges)
Prilocaine 3% plus felypressin 0·03 iu/ml	Effective analgesia for 90 minutes Methaemoglobinaemia in excess May be preferred for patients on tricyclic antidepressants[c]	600 mg (10 × 2-ml cartridges)
Bupivicaine 0·25% or 0·5%	Useful where long-acting LA is required (up to 8 hours)	2 mg/kg

[a] Allergy to local anaesthetic agents, if it exists, is *very* rare (supposed 'allergies' are common, however)
[b] The total dose of adrenaline must never exceed 500 μg, ie not more than 40 ml of a 1 in 80 000 solution.
[c] Although there is no good evidence that lignocaine with adrenaline is dangerous.

Potential airways obstruction
- Ludwig's angina
- Angioedema
- Hereditary angioedema
- Blood coagulation defects

Respiratory disease
- Including respiratory tract infections

Severe cardiovascular disease
- Ischaemic heart disease, including myocardial infarct in previous 2 years
- Hypertension

Severe anaemia
- Including sickle cell disease or trait

Metabolic disorders
- Liver disease
- Renal disease

Endocrinopathies

- Thyrotoxicosis
- Hypothyroidism
- Severe diabetes, especially if poorly controlled
- Addison's disease or adrenocortical suppression

Other conditions

- Cervical spine pathology, including involvement in Down's syndrome or rheumatoid arthritis
- Specific contra-indications to anaesthetic drugs, eg porphyria (see Tables 5.22–5.24)
- Pregnancy (see Section 3.10)
- Myopathies
- Disseminated sclerosis

Drug usage and recent previous general anaesthetics*

Particularly corticosteroids, anticoagulants, alcohol or narcotics (see Chapter 7 and Tables 5.22–5.24)

6.2 Conscious sedation

Assessment and selection of patients

It is important to determine:

What necessitates sedation?
Specific fears (eg of needles); past experiences (eg gagging problems).

Previous experience with sedation or general anaesthesia
Have there been problems?

Medical history
Any contra-indications to *sedation*, or are any special precautions indicated?

Social history
Can the patient bring a responsible escort if required to do so?
Is the patient able to take time off work?

---

*Repeated administration of halothane may produce 'halothane hepatitis'.

Whether the patient's responsibilities (eg their job, night duty, caring for young children) will permit them to receive sedation.

The patient's expectations
Initially, many nervous patients only want to be relieved of pain, but as their confidence in you grows, they may become more interested in what treatment is available.

Dental examination and radiographs
Dental examination may need to be carried out in a 'non-dental' chair with a pen torch and mouth mirror. Some patients will find intra-oral radiographs difficult to tolerate, so extra-oral radiographs may be more appropriate on the first visit.

Selection of sedation technique
Available are:
- Oral sedation, using a benzodiazepine such as diazepam or temazepam
- Inhalational sedation, using nitrous oxide and oxygen (relative analgesia). (Enflurane and isoflurane are currently under trial.)
- Intravenous sedation (IV sedation), using a benzodiazepine, usually midazolam (Hypnovel)

Inhalational sedation is preferred since it is more convenient for both operator and patient, and the drug can easily be withdrawn.

Legal aspects of sedation
In April 1978, a working party into the role of the dentist using sedation drew up the Wylie report, which stated:

> 'Our definition of a simple sedation technique is one in which the use of a drug or drugs produces a state of depression of the central nervous system enabling treatment to be carried out, but during which verbal contact with the patient is maintained throughout the period of sedation. The drugs and techniques used should carry a margin of safety wide enough to render unintended loss of consciousness unlikely.'

In 1983, the General Dental Council laid down recommendations in their Notice for the Guidance of Dentists.

> 'Where intravenous or inhalational sedation techniques are to be employed, a suitably experienced practitioner may assume the responsibility of sedation of the patient, as well as operating, provided that, as a minimum requirement, a second appropriate person is

present throughout. Such an appropriate person might be a suitably trained dental surgery assistant or ancillary dental worker, whose experience and training enables that person to be an efficient member of the dental team and is capable of monitoring the clinical condition of the patient. Should the occasion arise, he or she must also be capable of assisting the dentist in case of emergency.'

In 1988, the GDC added: 'Neither general anaesthesia nor sedation should be employed unless proper equipment for their administration and adequate facilities for the resuscitation of the patient are readily available, with both the operator and his/her staff trained in their use.'

It is extremely important that the DSA involved conforms to the definition of a *second appropriate person* and that you revise your emergency procedures with that person at regular and frequent intervals.

The 'second appropriate person' must be present throughout the treatment and must not leave the surgery at any time. Therefore, when patients are being sedated, a *third* person must be present to fetch things, carry out administrative duties and answer the phone.

Consent to sedation

(1) Explain fully exactly what is to be done at each visit; consent *must* be informed. This means that the patient must be given an explanation of the nature, purpose and effects of the procedure, and the balance of risks, appropriate to his or her intelligence and interest.
(2) Give written pre-operative and post-operative instructions.
(3) Get a consent form signed, giving permission for a sedation technique to be used together with local analgesia and consent for the operative procedure.

Oral sedation

Advantages
● Helpful for the moderately apprehensive patient, simple and relatively safe (Table 6.3).

Disadvantages
● Variability in absorption time for drugs taken by mouth (the patient may become sedated too soon, possibly endangering themselves en route to the surgery, or too late).
● Compliance of patient: may have the effect of making some children *hyperexcitable*, some children are rather resistant to diazepam. Elderly patients may be sensitive (Tables 5.16 and 5.17).

Table 6.3   Premediation of outpatients[a]

		Time	Route	Dose
Adult				
either	Temazepam[b]	0·5 to 1 hour pre-op	O[c]	10–30 mg
or	Diazepam	0·5 to 1 hour pre-op	O or IM	5–10 mg
Child	Diazepam	1·5 hours pre-op	O or IM or rectal	2 mg (or more according to age)

[a] Avoid the oral route if GA is to be given, unless the anaesthetist is content to have it given orally.
[b] More rapid onset, shorter action and less hangover than diazepam.
[c] Elixir, tablets or capsules. Absorption from soft gelatin capsules is quicker than from hard gelatin capsules or tablets.

Diazepam

Diazepam can either be taken as one dose (5–15 mg for an adult) one hour before treatment, or in divided doses (eg 5 mg the night before treatment, a further 5 mg on waking and another 5 mg one hour before treatment).

Temazepam

A dose of 30 mg temazepam taken one hour pre-operatively provides a level of sedation about the same as that seen with intravenous diazepam in lipid emulsion (Diazemuls).

Inhalation sedation (relative analgesia: RA)

Indications include:

- Anxiety.
- Marked gagging.
- Some casual patients.

Advantages

- Patient is conscious and cooperative.
- Non-invasive.
- The drug can be easily and rapidly altered or discontinued.
- Protective reflexes minimally impaired.
- The drug is administered and excreted through the lungs, and virtually total recovery takes place within the first 15 minutes of cessation of administration. The patient may, therefore, attend and leave the surgery or hospital unaccompanied.
- No strict fasting is required beforehand.
- A degree of analgesia (although LA is often still required).
- No hypotension or respiratory depression.

Disadvantages
- The level of sedation is largely dependent on psychological reassurance/back-up.
- The nitrous oxide must be administered continuously whilst required.
- Amnesia or a distortion of time may occur, but this may be advantageous.
- Nitrous oxide pollution of the surgery atmosphere. This can be reduced by:
  - (*a*) Scavenging equipment.
  - (*b*) Venting the suction machine outside the building.
  - (*c*) Minimising conversation from the patient.
  - (*d*) Testing the equipment weekly for leakage.
  - (*e*) Keeping the equipment well maintained with 6-monthly servicing.
  - (*f*) Ventilating the surgeries with fresh air (eg open window and door fan and open window air conditioning).
  - (*g*) Monitoring the air, eg Barnsley N_2O Monitor which can be obtained from:

    Dr O'Sullivan,
    Quality Control Pharmacist,
    Barnsley District General Hospital,
    Gamber Road, Barnsley S75 2EP

Contra-indications to relative analgesia

Psychological
Fear or non-acceptance of the nasal mask.

Medical
- Temporary (eg heavy cold) or permanent nasal obstruction (eg deviated nasal septum).
- Cyanosis at rest due to chronic cardiac (eg congenital disease) or respiratory disease (eg chronic bronchitis or emphysema). These patients are usually dependent on low O_2 levels for their respiratory drive.
- Severe psychiatric disease, where cooperation is not possible.
- Inability to communicate with the patient.
- First trimester of pregnancy.
- Some neuromuscular diseases (eg ischaemic heart disease, or severe anaemia).

Essential advice to the patient
On the day of treatment:
- DO eat as normal before treatment.

- DO take your routine medicines at the usual times.
- DON'T drink any alcohol.

After treatment:
The effects of the sedative gas normally wear off very quickly and you will be fit to go back to work or travel home. (Although recovery is very rapid and patients may be safely discharged without an escort, they should be discouraged from driving, particularly 2-wheeled vehicles, immediately after treatment.)

Procedure for relative analgesia
(1) Check relative analgesia machine is ready and working, that extra nitrous oxide and oxygen are available and that you are completely familiar with the machine. Use a scavenging system.

(2) Lie the patient comfortably supine in the chair with legs uncrossed, and the equipment as unobtrusive as possible.

(3) Explain the procedure to the patient.

(4) Allow O_2 to flow (eg 5 litres/minute for a small adult, 7 litres/minute for a large adult).

(5) Close the air entrainment port if present on the nasal mask.

(6) Ask the patient to place the facemask on to his/her nose. Adjust the mask and tubing to give a good fit.

(7) Warn the patient that the O_2 will feel cold.

(8) Check that the oxygen flow volume is adequate by:
   (*a*) Asking the patient if he/she is receiving the right amount of air (do not directly suggest too much or too little).

   (*b*) Watching whether the patient is mouth-breathing to supplement the flow.

   (*c*) Watching the reservoir bag to see if it is under or over inflating, in which case the flow is wrong.

(9) Adjust the rate of O_2 flow until a comfortable minute volume is achieved. The correct volume for each patient must be found at each visit.

(10) Now turn nitrous oxide flow to 10% (90% O_2), informing the patient that he may feel changes, such as a feeling of warmth, heaviness/ lightheadedness, tingling of hands and feet, a feeling of remoteness, a change in visual and auditory acuity.

The signs of inhalation sedation are positive and pleasant
- relaxation
- warmth
- tingling or numbness
- visual or auditory changes
- slurring of speech
- slowed responses, eg reduced frequency of blinking, delayed response to verbal instructions or questioning.

Maintain 10% N_2O for one full minute; continue the verbal reassurance at all times.

(11) Increase the N_2O flow with a minute-long increment of 10% N_2O (to a total of 20% N_2O) and then proceed in minute-long increments of 5% N_2O until the patient appears and feels quite relaxed, reiterating suggested sensation changes all the time.

Machine output flows of between 20% and 35% N_2O in O_2 commonly allow for a state of detached sedation and analgesia, without any loss of consciousness or danger of obtunded reflexes. At these levels, patients are aware of operative procedures and are cooperative without being fearful.

If the normal patient cannot maintain an open mouth then he is too deeply sedated. A possible exception may be in the case of a handicapped patient, unable to maintain an open mouth even without sedation. If a prop is then used, extra careful observation of the depth of sedation is essential.

If, after a period of relaxation, the patient becomes restless or apprehensive, this usually means the level of N_2O is too high and the percentage should be reduced to a more comfortable level. The patient can then be maintained at an appropriate level until the operative procedure (or that part of it which the patient does not normally tolerate) is completed.

(12) Give the LA injection.

(13) Monitor the patient throughout by checking the pulse and respiratory rate at frequent intervals. The patient should be conscious and able to respond when directed. Dozing is safe, but snoring indicates partial

airway obstruction and must be corrected immediately. Both operator and assistant should carefully monitor the patient.

(14) When the sedation is to be terminated, the N_2O flow is shut off, so that 100% O_2 is given for 2 full minutes to counteract possible diffusion hypoxia.

(15) Remove the facemask and slowly bring the patient upright over the next few minutes.

(16) The patient will usually be fit to leave after 15 minutes. Check that he/she is totally alert and well.

Intravenous sedation

Sedation with benzodiazepines (Table 6.4)

Intravenous administration of benzodiazepines produces:

- Acute detachment for 20–30 minutes and a state of relaxation for a further hour or so.
- Some anterograde amnesia for the same period.
- Minimal cardiovascular depression (a small degree of hypotension and bradycardia may simply be a relief of the hypertension and tachycardia of anxiety).

Midazolam (Hypnovel) is a benzodiazepine which is soluble in water and available in a 2-ml ampoule in a concentration of 5 mg/ml or in a 5-ml ampoule in a concentration of 2 mg/ml. Note that both presentations contain 10 mg midazolam in one ampoule.

Diazepam (Diazemuls and Valium) is another benzodiazepine, not water soluble, which is presented in a 2-ml ampoule in a concentration of 5 mg/ml for intravenous or intramuscular injections.

Midazolam is preferred because it is non-irritant in aqueous solution, has a much shorter half-life than diazepam, (in the region of 1–2 hours), no significant metabolites (so that recovery is both quicker and smoother) and has more predictable amnesic properties than diazepam.

Advantages

- Adequate level of sedation is attained pharmacologically rather than with psychological back-up.
- Amnesia removes unpleasant memories.
- The patient may take a light meal up to 2 hours before treatment.

Table 6.4 Benzodiazepines for intravenous sedation (see also Tables 5.22–5.24)[a]

Drug	Adult dose	Comments
Midazolam	0·07 mg/kg (up to 7·5 mg total dose)	Often preferred to diazepam because: (1) Onset of action is quicker (30–100 s) (2) Amnesia is more profound, starting 2–5 minutes after administration and lasting up to 40 minutes (with no retrograde amnesia) (3) Recovery is more rapid. Midazolam is virtually completely eliminated within 5–6 hours, without the recurrence of drowsiness which may follow the use of diazepam (4) Incidence of venous thrombosis is less (than with diazepam in organic solvent).
Diazepam in organic solvent	Up to 20 mg	Gives sedation with amnesia but no analgesia Give slowly IV in 2·5-mg increments until ptosis begins, ie eyelids begin to droop (Verril's sign). Rapid injection may cause respiratory depression. Then give local analgesia Disadvantages: (1) May cause pain or thrombophlebitis (2) Drowsiness returns transiently 4–6 hours post-operatively (due to metabolism to oxazepam and desmethyldiazepam) (3) May produce mild hypotension and respiratory depression
Diazepam as emulsion	Up to 20 mg	Preferred since, although it has most of the actions above, it causes less thrombophlebitis and therefore can be given into veins on dorsum of hand. Do not give intramuscularly.

[a]Particular caution in pregnancy, the elderly, children and those with liver or respiratory disease. Do *not* give pentazocine with a benzodiazepine.

Disadvantages

- Benzodiazepines produce no added analgesia, therefore LA is needed.
- Once administered, the drug cannot be 'discontinued' or 'switched off' (compare with RA).

- There is a short period after injection when direct laryngeal reflexes may be impaired and therefore a mouth sponge/gauze or rubber dam must be used to protect against accidental inhalation of water or debris.
- *Patient must be accompanied home from surgery and may not drive or work machinery, including domestic appliances, make important decisions, or drink alcohol for 24 hours.*

Contra-indications

Psychological:
- Frightened of needles and injections.

Social:
- Other responsibilities (eg, caring for young children, shift work, inability to bring an escort).

Medical:
- Previous reaction to IV agents or any benzodiazepine.
- Pregnancy (also, caution during breast feeding).
- Severe psychiatric disease.
- Alcohol or narcotic dependency (may render usual doses ineffective).
- Children: a considerable variability in reaction to diazepam has been noted in children and RA is the method of choice in most cases.
- Liver or kidney disease.
- Glaucoma.
- Potential drug interactions with (see Tables 5.22–5.24):

    (*a*) Cimetidine (for gastric ulceration)

    (*b*) Disulfiram (for treatment of alcoholism)

    (*c*) Drugs for Parkinsonism, eg levodopa.

    (*d*) Drugs which decrease cardiovascular and respiratory function, eg antihypertensive drugs, antihistamines, narcotic analgesics, hypnotics, sedatives and anti-epileptics.

It should be noted that these drug interactions are not necessarily absolute contra-indications to the careful use of intravenous or oral benzodiazepines.

Flumazenil

Flumazenil is an imidazobenzodiazepine – a specific benzodiazepine antagonist. It allows rapid reversal of conscious sedation with benzodiazepines by specific competitive inhibition for benzodiazepine receptors.

Dosage. Available as 5-ml ampoules containing 500 µg. Initial dose 200 µg (2 ml) over 15 seconds. If the desired level of consciousness is not obtained within 60 seconds, give 100 µg at 60-second intervals, up to a maximum of 1000 µg. Usual dose required: 300–600 µg.

Flumazenil has a short duration of action (half-life approx. 50 minutes); therefore, repeated doses may be required until all possible central effects of the benzodiazepines have subsided. If drowsiness recurs, an infusion of 100–400 µg/hour may be employed.

Contra-indications and warnings.
- Hypersensitivity to benzodiazepines and flumazenil.
- Pregnancy.
- Epilepsy.
- Impaired liver function (metabolised in liver).
- Use of psychotropic drugs (eg tricyclics).

Side-effects (rare).
- Flushing.
- Nausea/vomiting.
- Anxiety/palpitations/fear.
- Seizures.
- Transient rise in BP and pulse rate.

Overdosage. A dose of 100 mg given IV has caused no adverse reaction. Overdosage is therefore unlikely to occur.

Note: If patients are given flumazenil following IV sedation procedures, they must still follow the normal instructions given after sedation (ie no driving, operating machinery, etc).

6.3 Routine checks before out-patient general anaesthesia or intravenous sedation for dental treatment

- Patient's name and hospital number.
- Nature, side and site of operation.
- Medical and social history (Section 6.1), particularly of cardiorespiratory disease or bleeding tendency, and the availability of suitable social support on discharge.
- Consent has been obtained in writing from the patient or, in a person under 16 years of age, from a parent/guardian, and that the patient

adequately understands the nature of the operation and sequelae (see Section 6.2).

- Necessary investigations (eg radiographs) are available.
- Patient has had *nothing* by mouth for *at least* the previous 4 hours.
- Patient has emptied bladder.
- Patient's dentures* have been removed and bridges, crowns and loose teeth have been noted by the anaesthetist.
- Necessary premedication (and, where indicated, regular medication (eg the contraceptive pill, anticonvulsants or antidepressants) have been given (see Table 6.5 and Sections 3.4 and 3.5 concerning steroid therapy and diabetes).
- Anaesthetic and suction apparatus are working satisfactorily, correct drugs are available and drug expiry date has not passed. Emergency kit and flumazenil available.
- Patient will be escorted by a responsible adult.
- Patient has been warned not to drive, operate machinery, drink alcohol or make important decisions for 24 hours post-operatively.

Special points related to particular techniques are outlined below.

Avoid acting as operator–anaesthetist: have a third party present.

Before operation

Check the identity of the patient. Ask the patient his/her name. Also, ensure that the teeth marked for extraction agree with those entered in:

- the consent form.
- the patient's notes.
- the referring practitioner's notes.

Any discrepancy must be investigated, if necessary by conferring with the clinician who signed the consent form.

- Check that any relevant medical history is drawn to the anaesthetist's attention.
- Ensure that the consent form has been signed by the patient/parent/ guardian and a clinician (member of staff).
- In the case of removal of permanent teeth, check that radiographs showing the complete root structure are available.

At operation

Wear disposable rubber gloves. It is accepted that a strict 'no-touch' technique is not possible. However, once the operator's gloves have become contaminated with the patient's saliva and/or blood, he/she will

---

*Or other oral appliances.

touch only the work surface of the paper cover of the trolley and the instruments or materials used for the operation.

After operation

The case notes and day book *must* be completed, dated and signed by the responsible member of clinical staff. In hospital, the notes and day book must be countersigned by the supervising senior member of staff.

See the patient (and parents) before discharge. Consider whether analgesics and/or antibiotics need to be prescribed.

Special precautions in addition to routine checks in Section 6.2

- Treat fit individuals only (Section 6.1) and take particular note of respiratory disease.
- Have the patient lying horizontal.

Procedure for intravenous sedation

(1) Select a suitable site in the antecubital fossa (or dorsum of the hand) for venepuncture. A green needle is usually used, but an indwelling needle of the Butterfly type can be used so that a patent vein can be maintained throughout the procedure. The arm should be kept straight with a board if the antecubital fossa is used.

(2) Occlude the venous return above the elbow with a tourniquet, or ask an assistant to squeeze the arm. Alternatively, place the tourniquet above the wrist to use the back of the hand.

(3) Cleanse the skin with a suitable antiseptic (eg isopropanol 70% or chlorhexidine 0·5%). Select the most readily palpable vein which is remote from the brachial artery.

(4) Unless a Butterfly needle is used, bend the needle by about 30°, so that it can be placed flat on the skin, bevel upwards, without obstruction from the needle hub or syringe barrel. Tap the vein until it becomes reflexly dilated, tense the skin with one hand distal to the chosen puncture site. Place the needle flat on the skin and press downwards. Slide the needle smoothly along the skin and it will pierce the surface and enter the vein easily. Once through the skin, which is the most painful part of the procedure, the needle can be manipulated so that the technique of entering a vein from the side could be used. Advance the needle until two thirds of its length is within the vein. The appearance of blood within the tubing on aspiration confirms correct positioning.

(5) Secure the needle or Butterfly needle with non-allergenic tape.

(6) Give a very small intravenous 'first dose', to ensure that the needle is in a vein and that there is no adverse reaction (Table 6.5).

(7) Slowly inject the prepared drug, warning the patient of a possible cold sensation at the needle site or as the drug tracks up the arm. Provided one is sure that the needle is correctly positioned, the patient should be reassured that this sensation will pass within a short period of time. Stop injecting if pain is felt, eg radiating down the forearm, indicating entry into an artery. Inject 3 mg midazolam over 30 seconds, then pause for a further 90 seconds. In young or middle-aged adults, *much smaller* doses are necessary than in older patients. Give further increments of 1 mg (0·5 ml) every 30 seconds, until sedation is judged to be adequate. Watch for any adverse responses and particularly any respiratory impairment.

The correct dose has been given when there is slurring of speech and the patient is relaxed. Ptosis is not a reliable end point; adequate sedation with midazolam may occur before ptosis is evident.

(8) Give LA.

(9) Protect the airway, especially in conservation procedures, ie use rubber dam, butterfly sponges, etc.

(10) Protect the patient's eyes during operation.

(11) Operative procedures may be started after a couple of minutes. Approximately 30 minutes of sedation time is available for the operator. Since there may be considerable muscle relaxation, a prop may be needed to maintain the mouth open. *The airway must be protected because the laryngeal reflexes are obtunded after the administration of intravenous drugs, and eye protection must be used.* A barrier to prevent accidental inhalation of debris must be used, and this may be rubber dam, butterfly sponge or a gauze square. Some advocate the use of a small dose of either hyoscine or atropine in addition to benzodiazepines to reduce the risks arising from excessive salivation or bronchial secretion, but the advantages gained are outweighed by the discomfort of a very dry mouth and the potential dangers of using atropinics.

(12) Monitor the patient frequently by means of the pulse, respiratory rate and the patient's colour. The patient should remain conscious and able to respond when directed.

(13) At the end of the procedure, slowly bring the patient upright over 5 minutes. The patient should recover over at least another 15 minutes, under the direct supervision of a member of the dental team or his escort.

Table 6.5 Complications of intravenous injections[a]

Complication	Cause	Treatment
Haematoma	Leakage of blood, because of inadequate pressure on vein after needle removed. Mainly occurs from dorsum of hand veins	Avoid by using antecubital veins and applying firm pressure
Extravenous injection	Needle moves during injection. Mainly causes problems with thiopentone and diazepam (Valium)	Inject normal saline (or plain lignocaine 2%) at site
Intra-arterial injection	Ensure that the blood vessel is not pulsating before injecting. Main problem is with thiopentone	Inject plain lignocaine 2% (5 ml). Call for medical assistance
Venous thrombosis	Viscous or irritant solutions injected into small veins. Main problems are with thiopentone, diazepam (Valium)	Icthammol in glycerin application. Analgesics. Rest. Plus antibiotics if not resolved in 7 days

[a]Any of these may be the cause of pain.

(14) The patient must not be discharged until at least one hour has elapsed since the drug was given.

(15) The patient should be discharged into the care of his/her escort and instructed that he/she should rest quietly at home for the remainder of the day and refrain from driving or operating machinery or making important decisions for 24 hours. Post-operative instructions together with any pertaining to the dentistry performed should be given on a written sheet for the patient to refer to later, as he may still be under the effects of the amnesic properties of the drug.

Advice to patients after dental surgery under out-patient general anaesthetics or intravenous sedation

Give verbal *and* written instructions along the following lines:
Some of the effects of the anaesthetic will last for the rest of the day; therefore, bring a responsible escort, do not eat or drink anything before operation. For the next 24 hours, you must not:

- Drink alcohol
- Ride a bicycle, or drive any vehicle
- Operate machinery at work or in your own home

- Go to work or do housework or cooking
- Undertake any responsible business matters or sign important documents

After a tooth has been extracted, the socket will usually bleed for a short time. The bleeding stops because of the formation of a healthy clot of blood in the tooth socket. These clots are easily disturbed and, if this happens, more bleeding will occur. To avoid disturbances of the clot, please follow this advice:

- After leaving the hospital, do not rinse out your mouth for 24 hours.
- Do not disturb the clot in the socket with your tongue or fingers.
- For the rest of the day, take only food which requires no chewing.
- Do not chew on the affected side for at least 3 days. If both sides of your mouth are involved, you should have a soft diet for 3 days.
- Avoid hot drinks, hot baths, alcohol, exercise, unnecessary talking or excitement, sitting in front of a fire or in overheated rooms.

If the tooth socket continues to bleed after you have left the hospital, do not be alarmed; much of the liquid which appears to be blood is saliva.

Make a small pad from a clean handkerchief or cotton wool, place it directly over the socket and close the teeth firmly on it. Keep up the pressure for 15–30 minutes. If the bleeding still does not stop, seek advice from the hospital or the resident dental surgeon.

6.4 Muscle relaxants

Muscle relaxants are used during the induction of GA, to allow laryngeal relaxation, in order to permit intubation, and also to relax the jaw and various muscles. *Patients must then be ventilated.*

Suxamethonium

- A depolarising muscle relaxant.
- Effect appears within 1 minute and persists for 5 minutes.
- Respiration must be assisted as the patient is paralysed and unable to breathe.
- Recovery is rapid; drug reversal is not feasible.
- Side-effects: muscle pain and hypertension.
- Contra-indicated particularly in suxamethonium sensitivity (pseudocholinesterase deficiency), malignant hyperthermia, and fascial space infections (eg Ludwig's angina) (see Tables 5.22–5.24).

Tubocurarine

- Non-depolarising muscle relaxant.
- Effect appears within 3 minutes and persists for 40 minutes.
- Respiration must be assisted.
- Anticholinesterases such as neostigmine can reverse the paralysis.
- Side-effects: hypotension, facial flushing and bronchospasm because of histamine release.

Other agents

Pancuronium, atracuronium and vecuronium are newer non-depolarising muscle relaxants, which produce less histamine release than tubocurarine and are more popular.

6.5 Gaseous anaesthetics

Table 6.6 Gaseous anaesthetics[a] (see also Tables 5.22–5.24)

Drug	Comments
Nitrous oxide[b]	Analgesic, but weak anaesthetic. Non-explosive. No cardiorespiratory effects. Mainly used as a vehicle for other anaesthetic agents. Abuse or prolonged occupational exposure can cause megaloblastic anaemia.
Halothane[c]	The most widely used anaesthetic agent. Non-explosive. Anaesthetic but weak analgesic. Causes fall in BP, cardiac dysrrhythmias and bradycardia (avoid adrenaline-containing LA). Hepatotoxic on repeated administration. Post-anaesthetic shivering is common, vomiting rare
Enflurane	Less effective anaesthesia than halothane. Non-explosive. Less likely to produce dysrrhythmias or affect liver than halothane. Powerful cardiorespiratory depressant. Contra-indicated in epileptics
Isoflurane	Isomer of enflurane but more potent. Causes less cardiac but more respiratory depression than halothane. Muscle relaxant.
Trichloroethylene[d]	Analgesic and anaesthetic. Non-explosive. Bradycardia and dysrrhythmias are common as are tachypnoea; causes nausea and vomiting

[a] Gas scavenging should be used.
[b] Abuse may lead to disturbed vitamin B12 metabolism, megaloblastosis, and neurological sequelae.
[c] Do not give halothane if patient has had halothane within the previous 12 weeks or has previously had an adverse reaction to halothane.
[d] Rarely used because of slow induction and long recovery.

Table 6.7 Management of general anaesthesia in patients on regular medication

Drug	Action
Antidepressants, eg MAOI, tricyclics	Consult physician and, where possible, stop for 2 weeks before GA
Antidiabetic drugs	Omit morning dose (see Section 3.5)
Anti-epileptic drugs	Continue as normal up to and after GA. Avoid methohexitone
Antihypertensives	Particular care to ensure that hypotension does not occur with or after GA
Bronchodilators, eg aminophylline, isoprenaline	Continue medication, but care with halothane (danger of cardiac arrhythmias)
Cardiac glycosides, eg digoxin	Continue as normal up to and after GA but care with suxamethonium (danger of cardiac arrhythmias)
Cytotoxic drugs	Avoid suxamethonium (prolonged respiratory paralysis)
Lithium	Omit before *major* surgery (risk of lithium intoxication)
Oral contraceptives	Continue as normal up to and after GA[a]
Sedatives and tranquillisers, eg chlorpromazine, promethazine	Consult physician and, where possible, stop drug before GA. Otherwise reduced dose of GA indicated (danger of hypotension and enhanced respiratory depression)
Various: fenfluramine, L-Dopa	Consult physician and where possible, stop 12 hours before GA (danger of cardiac arrhythmias)

[a]Unless there is a danger of thromboembolism.

6.6 Intravenous anaesthetics

Table 6.8   Intravenous anaesthetics[a] (see also Tables 5.22–5.24)

Drug	Adult induction dose	Comments
Etomidate	0·2 mg/kg	Good for outpatient anaesthesia. Pain on injection: use large vein and give fentanyl 200 μg first. After operation, give naloxone 0·1–0·2 mg and oxygen. Little cardiovascular effect. Often involuntary movements, cough and hiccup. Hepatic metabolism. Avoid in traumatised patient, as may suppress adrenal steroid production
Ketamine	1–2 mg/kg	Rise in BP, cardiac rate, intra-ocular pressure. Little respiratory depression. Often hallucinations. Contra-indicated in hypertension, cerebrovascular or ocular disorders. Rarely used in dentistry
Methohexitone	1·5 mg/kg 1% solution (10 mg/ml)	Ultra short-acting barbiturate. The most commonly used IV anaesthetic in dentistry. No analgesia. Mild hyperventilation or apnoea if given rapidly. Dose-dependent cardiovascular depression. Danger of laryngospasm. Relatively non-irritant to tissues. Hepatic metabolism. Contra-indicated in: epilepsy, cardiorespiratory disease, porphyria, barbiturate sensitivity. Rare: acute allergy, cough, hiccups, sneeze
Thiopentone	2·5 mg/kg (use 2·5% solution)	Ultra short-acting barbiturate. No analgesia. Rapid injection may cause apnoea. Dose-dependent cardiorespiratory depression. Irritant to tissues. Hepatic metabolism. Contra-indicated in cardiorespiratory disease, liver disease, porphyria
Propofol	2–2·5 mg/kg	Sometimes pain on injection. Rapid recovery

[a]Particular caution in pregnancy, the elderly, children and those with liver or respiratory disease.

7

Management of Patients Undergoing Surgical Procedures

Surgery should never be undertaken lightly. The possible benefits must be weighed against the risks and should always be discussed with the patient. The surgery must be carried out by a person with the appropriate expertise.

7.1 Indications for in-patient treatment and admission to hospital

Examples of indications for routine admission for in-patient care

Major operations
- Orthognathic surgery.
- Cancer surgery.
- Fracture surgery.
- Some preprosthetic and orthodontic surgery.
- Surgery involving extensive vascular lesions.
- Multiple or complicated extractions.

Systemic disease
- Which may influence anaesthesia (eg cardiorespiratory disease, sickle cell anaemia).
- Which may directly influence surgery (eg bleeding disorder).
- Which may influence dental treatment indirectly (eg occasionally where treatment might otherwise necessitate multiple courses of antibiotics for cover against infective endocarditis).
- Some immunocompromised patients.

Investigations
- Complicated investigations.

Social reasons
- Some psychiatric patients.
- Some handicapped patients.
- Patients living alone or far from medical care.

Others
- Complicated medical treatment.
- Patient having difficulty eating.

Examples of indications for urgent admission to hospital
Trauma
- Middle facial third fractures.
- Mandibular fractures unless simple and undisplaced.
- Zygomatic fractures where there is danger of ocular damage.
- Laryngeal trauma.
- Head injury (see Chapter 8) and cervical spine injury.
- Other serious injuries.
- Patients in shock.
- Loss of consciousness

Inflammatory lesions and infections
- Cervical fascial space infection.
- Oral infections when patient is 'toxic' (see Table 1.7).
- Tuberculosis (some).
- Severe viral infections.
- Severe vesiculo-bullous disorders (pemphigus and Stevens–Johnson syndrome).

Blood loss
- Severe or persistent haemorrhage (particularly in patients with a bleeding tendency).
- Bleeding, highly anxious patients.

Others
- Airway obstruction.
- Disturbed, severely depressed or some other psychiatric patients.
- Battered babies.
- Diabetics out of control because of oral pain or infection.

Always discuss the case with the senior or delegated member of staff who is responsible for that session.

7.2 Admission of patients to hospital

The responsible consultant, or his deputy, must be informed if a patient is admitted under his care, and the bed bureau and the relevant ward sister must be told.

Patients' reactions to hospitalisation and illness

Patients admitted as emergencies may be acutely ill and often disturbed by an ambulance journey. Many who have been on the routine waiting list feel fine and come to hospital knowing that, in the next few days, they have before them discomfort and perhaps danger. Their routine has been upset; they have left the security and privacy of their homes and the comfort of relatives for an alien world which they may regard with fear. They feel vulnerable and at a disadvantage.

The most normal and self-sufficient individual will find these circumstances daunting; the old, the handicapped and the very young may well be overwhelmed and become distressed. Patients of different ethnic backgrounds also vary in their emotional response to illness, pain, operation or hospitalisation.

An operation is a new and forbidding prospect to most patients. The idea that patients are happier if they do not know what is planned for them is nonsense; they are entitled to be told what is going to happen to them. The difficulty about talking to patients is how to explain things without frightening and confusing them. However, it is probably better to risk this than to have an apprehensive patient complaining about the secrecy of his surgeon. Most patients, although not interested in technical details, require a simple explanation and reassurance.

Relatives

Relatives are usually interested and concerned, although occasionally intrusive or abusive. Do not forget the question of confidentiality (see Section 1.7) but, with this in mind, the date and time of operation and discharge may well be needed by caring relatives. Speak personally to the relatives at a pre-arranged visit by them. Phone calls from relatives should be handled by the nursing staff in the first instance. Try and avoid being bleeped (or paged) by relatives. Be careful and tactful in what you say.

7.3 Clerking, examination, investigations and consent

Clerking

Patients must be clerked on the day of admission. Do not allow unclerked patients to be on the ward for more than a short time (an hour or so, at most).

Patients with a positive recent history of contact with a communicable disease should not be admitted unless there is a good indication.

Examination

Patients with a proven diagnosis admitted for operation, should be examined specifically to confirm oral findings, for their fitness for a general anaesthetic, and for their ability to withstand the operative procedure.

Investigations (see also Chapter 1)

All patients admitted for a general anaesthetic should have estimations of haemoglobin, blood pressure and urinalysis.

Patients of over 50 years of age and any patient with a history of heart disease should have an electrocardiogram read. A chest radiograph may be indicated, particularly if there is respiratory disease. Liver function tests may be indicated if there is any suggestion of high alcohol intake.

Special investigations such as SickleDex test or HB_sAg screen may be indicated.

Consent (see Section 6.2)

Patients having operations must give informed consent in writing. In particular, they must be warned of possible adverse effects, about pre-operative preparation and about post-operative sequelae (eg pain), where they will be during their recovery, and the likely length of their stay in the clinic or hospital. Some units use written forms to help inform the patient, such as the one shown on page 189.

7.4 Pre-operative preparation, organising operating lists, and premedication

The day of admission

Patients are best admitted on the day before operation unless there are special pre-operative preparations or treatment to be carried out. They should be admitted early enough for the consultant to see them on his ward round before operation and the usual practice is for the houseman to draw up a tentative operating list which can be approved or rearranged by his seniors. Always clerk the patient in on the day of admission.

Removal of wisdom teeth

Dear Patient

As you know, we feel that your wisdom teeth should be removed. Here is some information which we hope will answer some of your questions.

Wisdom tooth removal is often necessary because of infection (which causes pain and swelling), decay, serious gum disease, the development of a cyst or because teeth are overcrowded. Wisdom teeth are removed under local anaesthetic (injection in the mouth), sedation or general anaesthetic in hospital, depending on your preference, the number of teeth to be removed and the difficulty of removal.

It is often necessary to make a small incision in the gum which is stitched afterwards. After removal of the teeth, your mouth will be sore and swollen and mouth movements will usually be stiff. Slight bleeding is also very common. These symptoms are quite normal, but can be expected to improve rapidly during the first week. It is quite normal for some stiffness and slight soreness to persist for two to three weeks. Pain and discomfort can be controlled with ordinary pain killers, such as paracetamol, and you might be prescribed antibiotic tablets. A dentist will be available to see you afterwards if you are worried, and will always want to check that healing is satisfactory.

Complications are rare, but occasionally wisdom tooth sockets become infected, when pain, swelling and stiffness will last longer than normal. About one in every ten patients suffers from this. About one in every twenty patients suffers from tingling or numbness of their lower lip or tongue after lower wisdom tooth removal. This is because nerves to these areas pass very close to the wisdom teeth and are occasionally bruised or damaged. This numbness nearly always disappears after about one month, but very occasionally lasts for a year or more.

Please let us know if we can give you any more information.

Points to remember:

- Patients in hospital in a strange environment may well benefit from a hypnotic the night before the operation (Table 5.16).
- Reassure patients (and relatives) about the various pre-operative and post-operative procedures, particularly if they are to recover in a strange ward, such as intensive care, or if they are to have nasogastric tubes, haloes, IV infusions, catheters, etc.
- Obtain informed consent to the operation. Record in writing when the warnings about possible complications have been given.
- Inform the anaesthetist of any relevant medical history (Section 6.1) and courteously enquire if he/she wishes to adopt any special measures or requires any investigations.
- Organise any required general or oral investigations.
- If there is any chance of severe haemorrhage, such as in major surgical procedures or patients with a bleeding tendency, take blood for grouping and cross-matching. Order blood if needed.
- Carry out any necessary pre-operative dental procedures (eg impressions), and arrange for necessary dental items to be in theatre on the day of operation.
- Warn the radiographers if radiographs will be required during operation.
- Warn the pathologists if a frozen section will be required; fill out the necessary request forms before the operation
- Warn the photographer if he will be required.
- Check that there is suitable social support for the patient on discharge.
- Tell the patient and relatives when the operation will take place, and roughly how long it will take to recover.

Regular theatre list
The order of patients for operation is decided on certain considerations:

(1) 'Big' cases should be done first.
(2) Patients with diabetes and highly anxious patients should be done early in the day.
(3) 'Dirty' cases (eg, opening an abscess) or 'hepatitis risk' or AIDS patients should be done last of all.
(4) 'Day cases' should be dealt with before 3.00 pm.
(5) The surgeon's preference.

The list should not be made too long. Time must be allowed for the induction of anaesthesia (usually about 15 minutes per patient) and for breaks.

The list should note:

(1) The name of the operator and responsible consultant;
(2) The start time;
(3) The theatre venue;
(4) The patient's name, hospital number, ward, operation and type of anaesthetic and should be sent to the theatre, ward, anaesthetist and surgeon. If the order of the list changes, all should be informed – including the patient and relatives.

The day of operation

Always check:

- the patient's name (and hospital number);
- the nature, side, and site of operation;
- the medical history (Section 6.1), particularly of cardiorespiratory disease or bleeding tendency;
- that consent has been obtained in writing from the patient or, in a person under 16 years of age, from a parent/guardian, and that the patient adequately understands the nature of the operation and sequelae;
- that necessary dental items such as splints, radiographs, and models are available;
- that the patient has had nothing by mouth for at least the previous 4 hours;
- that the patient has an empty bladder;
- that the patient has removed contact lenses;
- that the patient's dentures have been removed and bridges, crowns and loose teeth have been noted by the anaesthetist;
- that necessary premedication (and, where indicated, regular medication such as the contraceptive pill, anticonvulsants or antidepressants) has been given (see Chapter 6 and Sections 3.4 and 3.5 concerning steroid therapy and diabetes);
- that any blood, etc, that is needed has been arranged.

Give the necessary information to all involved in the patient's care, and ensure that the ward, consultant, theatre, and anaesthetist (if the patient is returning to a different ward, also inform the new ward and relatives) are given the following information:

Patient's details
- Name
- Hospital number

- Date of birth
- Sex
- Relevant medical history
- Ward

Surgical procedure
- Type of procedure
- Any special requirements
- Surgeon's and anaesthetist's name
- Time of operation
- Intended disposal of patient (back to ward, to intensive care or elsewhere)
- Special post-operative nursing requirements

Premedication (Tables 7.1 and 7.2)
Premedication details should be arranged with anaesthetist and ward sister.

The objects of premedication (premed) are:

- to allay anxiety;
- to reduce cardiac excitability;
- to reduce bronchial secretions;
- to provide some analgesia;
- to aid the induction of anaesthesia;
- to provide some amnesia.

Table 7.1   In-patient child pre-operative medication (see also Chapter 5)

Alternative drugs	Time before operation	Route	Dose
Trimeprazine	1·5 hours	O or IM	2–4 mg/kg body wt
Promethazine	1·5 hours	O or IM	2–3 mg/kg body wt
Atropine	0·5 to 1 hour	IM or SC	0·3 mg up to age 6 months 0·4 mg at 6 months to 2 years 0·6 mg if over 2 years of age
Diazepam	1·5 hours	O, IM or rectal	Up to 3 years give 1–5 mg Over 3 years give 5–10 mg

Table 7.2 In-patient adult perioperative medication (see also Chapter 5)

	Timing	Route	Dose
Night sedation			
(See Table 5.16)			
Premedication			
(1) Fit adults under age 65 years, *either*			
(a) Omnopon (papaveretum)	0·5–1 hour pre-operatively	IM or SC	10–20 mg
plus Scopolamine[a] (hyoscine)	0·5–1 hour pre-operatively	IM or SC	0·1–0·4 mg
or (b) Morphine	0·5–1 hour pre-operatively	IM or SC	10–15 mg
plus Atropine[a]	0·5–1 hour pre-operatively	IM or SC	0·6–0·75 mg
or (c) Temazepam	0·5–1 hour pre-operatively	O	10 mg
plus Metoclopramide[b]	0·5–1 hour pre-operatively	O	10 mg
(2) Ill adults or those between 65 and 80 years			
Morphine	0·5–1 hour pre-operatively	IM or SC	10 mg
plus Atropine[a]	0·5–1 hour pre-operatively	IM or SC	0·6 mg
(3) Very ill adults or those over 80 years			
atropine[a]	0·5–1 hour pre-operatively	IM or SC	0·6 mg
Anti-emetics			
Metoclopramide[b]	4–6-hourly	IM or O	5–10 mg
or Perphenazine	4–6-hourly	IM or O	2·5–5 mg
or Prochlorperazine	6-hourly	IM or O	12·5 mg
Post-operative analgesia			
Severe pain: Omnopon (papaveretum)	4–6-hourly	IM	10 mg
Moderate pain: codeine	4–6-hourly	O or IM	30 mg
Mild pain:			
Aspirin	6-hourly	O	300–600 mg
or Paracetamol	6-hourly	O	500–1000 mg

[a]Glycopyrronium bromide 4–5 µg/kg body weight IM or IV may be preferred as it produces control of salivary secretions with little effect on heart rate.
[b]Avoid metoclopramide in those under the age of 20 years, because of dystonic reactions.

Problems of cardiac rhythm irregularities are most common in infants and young children, and most children under the age of 12 years require premedication before in-patient general anaesthesia (Table 7.1).

The anaesthetist usually accepts responsibility for premedication and often has his own regime. Establish the protocol which the anaesthetist wishes you to follow. Do not be surprised at how one anaesthetist differs from another.

Timing of premedication

Atropine IM takes effect within 30 minutes; morphine takes about 1 hour, and premedication is effective for about 4 hours. Therefore, do not give premedication too early. If the operation is delayed for over 3 hours, repeat only the dose of atropine.

Do not give premedication too late; if there is not 30–60 minutes available before the operation, leave the anaesthetist to give suitable drugs intravenously.

Contra-indications and adverse reactions

Atropine is contra-indicated in glaucoma. It may also cause drowsiness, blurred vision, urine retention and dry mouth.

Hyoscine may cause the above effects as well as confusion; it should therefore be avoided in the elderly.

Morphine is contra-indicated in patients who have a head injury or respiratory disorders (see Section 5.5, and Tables 5.22–5.24).

Diazepam is contra-indicated in glaucoma and respiratory disorders.

Other preparations in major cases

Put up an intravenous infusion (5% dextrose at the rate of 2–3 litres/24 hours), so that there is ready access to a vein if transfusion should be needed.

Maxillofacial and orthognathic surgery (see also Section 9.7)

In addition to the checks needed before in-patient dental treatment under general anaesthesia, the following are required pre-operatively.

- Ensure that the patient and relatives are made aware that the patient may awake post-operatively
  - (*a*) in the intensive care unit;
  - (*b*) with fixation;
  - (*c*) with intravenous cannulae, nasal tubes, etc;
  - (*d*) sometimes with hair shaved and facial sutures.
- A chest radiograph should be taken; the anaesthetic is likely to be

prolonged and a radiograph is useful as a baseline if there are post-operative complications.

- Blood group and cross-match 2 pints (or more) (Table 7.14).
- Urea and electrolytes.
- Investigations relevant to the surgical procedure
  (a) Radiographs (and tracings);
  (b) Photographs;
  (c) Models and templates.
- Fixation, eg interdental wires, silver cap splints, fixed appliances, arch bars, Champey plates. Try in the splints where possible and cement with black copper cement where appropriate.
- Ensure that a bed is booked in intensive care and that the nursing staff are conversant with the post-operative management.
- Discuss the case with the anaesthetist.

Summary of checks before in-patient dental treatment under GA

Always check:

(a) the patient's name (and hospital number);
(b) the nature, side and site of operation;
(c) the medical history (Section 6.1) – *particularly* of cardiorespiratory disease or bleeding tendency;
(d) that consent has been obtained in writing from the patient or, in a person under 16 years of age, from a parent/guardian, and that the patient and, where appropriate, the relatives adequately understand the nature of the operation and sequelae (record this in writing);
(e) that necessary dental items (eg plates, splints, tracings, models, and radiographs) are available in the correct theatre;
(f) that the patient has had *nothing* by mouth for *at least* the previous 4 hours;
(g) that the patient has an empty bladder;
(h) that the patient's dentures have been removed and bridges, crowns and loose teeth have been noted by the anaesthetist;
(i) that necessary premedication (and, where indicated, regular medication such as the contraceptive pill, anticonvulsants or antidepressants) has been given, but not within the previous 4 hours.

In addition ensure that:

(a) the theatre is booked (and any unusual equipment prepared);
(b) the consultant surgeon and anaesthetist are informed;

(c) the treatment plan is organised;

(d) a haemoglobin estimation is done (particularly in patients 50 years and older, and those with cardiac or respiratory disease);

(e) chest radiographs taken;

(f) electrocardiogram (50 years and older or cardiorespiratory disease);

(g) blood grouped and cross-matched (if indicated; Section 7.10);

(h) urinalysis;

(i) urea and electrolytes;

(j) intensive care bed booked (if indicated).

7.5 Surgical operations: safeguards

Operating on the wrong patient

Causes

- Notes attached to the wrong patient following emergency admission.
- Rearrangement of beds in the ward on day of operation.
- Last-minute changes in theatre lists.
- Lack of care.

Precautions

All unconscious patients admitted through the accident department should be labelled (in the correct manner) before being taken to the ward. The label should bear the patient's surname, forenames and accident or in-patient number. Labelling the patient should be the responsibility of the accident sister or her deputy, or, at night, by the nurse-in-charge or her deputy. The surgeon or accident officer should see that unconscious patients are escorted by a nurse to the ward or theatre.

The dental surgeon who is to operate should check the patient before operation, check that the medical or dental record relates to the patient and *ask* the patient his name and the operation he is to have.

The anaesthetist should check that the medical record relates to the patient. The ward sister or deputy (or occasionally the accident sister) should label all patients by surname in full, forenames, and hospital number immediately before they are sent to the theatre.

The operations list should carry the patient's surname in full, forenames, hospital number, and the operation planned. The list should be displayed in the surgery or theatre, in the anaesthetic room, and in every ward which has a patient on the list or is to receive a patient from the list.

When sending from theatre for a patient:

(a) The theatre porter should bring a slip bearing the surname, forenames and number of the patient, or the patient's full name and number should be quoted over the telephone.

(b) The ward sister or her deputy should be responsible for seeing that the correct patient is sent to theatre, the patient has signed a consent form, the patient has received the prescribed premedications, where appropriate, the side of operation has been marked, and that the correct records and radiographs accompany the patient.

(c) In theatre, the theatre superintendent or deputy should be responsible for sending for patients.

Day-patients for minor operations and out-patients for any operation under general anaesthetic should be labelled in the same way as in-patients. Patients should have one hospital number, which should *always* be quoted on every paper. Children should be labelled with a plastic identification bracelet on admission to the ward. The utmost care should be taken in transcribing case histories from relatives.

Operating on the wrong side or area
Causes
- Wrong information or case papers. Wrong radiographs.
- Illegible case papers.
- Abbreviation of the words 'right' and 'left', or mistakes in dental charting.
- Failure to check the entry on the operating lists against the notes in theatre, together with the wrong case papers or the preparation of the wrong side or area.
- No routine procedure for marking operation side.
- Lack of care.

Precautions
The house surgeon should mark the side or area with an indelible skin pencil before the patient is sent to theatre. Before emergency operations, the surgeon should see the patient. The surgeon who decided upon the operation in the case of a patient going directly from the accident department to theatre should be responsible for marking the side or area.

Sisters should inform the operating surgeon if they find that a patient due to be sent to theatre has not been marked, but they should not undertake the marking themselves.

The words RIGHT and LEFT should always be written in full and in block letters. It is the responsibility of the dentist who explains the operation to witness the patient signing the correct consent form.

7.6 In theatre

Before scrubbing and gowning, ensure that last minute jobs have been done, such as checking that everything for theatre is ready, and that all necessary phone calls are made. Know your glove size.

Scrubbing-up and gowning

The essential points are:

(1) Lather the hands and forearms with soap or a special solution (Table 7.3).
(2) Scrub with a brush for 1 minute, especially the nails and hands. Vigorous scrubbing is open to the criticism that bacteria may be brought out of skin pores and increase rather than reduce skin bacterial counts.
(3) Lather and rinse hands and forearms vigorously for a further 5 minutes: turn taps on with elbows.
(4) Rinse off soap. Hold your hands up at a higher level than the elbows.
(5) Dry with a sterile towel. It is important to prevent the towel touching unsterile skin at the elbow and then wiping the opposite hand with it – very easy to do.
(6) The sterile gown is unfolded and the arms pushed into the armholes and then the arms are held up. A nurse should then pull down the shoulders and body of the gown and tie it behind. It is inadvisable to pull the sleeves up yourself because of the risk of inadvertently touching the mask or collar.
(7) Gloves are donned, care being taken not to touch the outside of the rubber with the skin of the opposite hand.
(8) Thereafter, observe a 'no touch' technique.

Preparing the patient

Painting-up

The operation site and several inches around in all directions should be painted with an antiseptic, dried with a sterile swab and then painted with a bactericidal agent. The eyelids should be carefully closed by the anaesthetist and covered with gauze pads, smeared with a little Vaseline, and secured with Sellotape, micropore or strapping. Some centres also use plastic or other eye-guards. One per cent Cetavlon solution is most suitable for preparing the face. It is not essential to paint inside the lips and mouth prior to oral surgery, although some do.

Spirit solutions must not be used to prepare the skin around the eyes.

Table 7.3   Hand washing

Agents	Comments
Chlorhexidine 4% + detergent	First choice for pre-operative preparation
Chlorhexidine 0·52% + alcohol + skin emollient	Where detergent cannot be used. Where hand basin not available
Povidone–iodine 7·5% + detergent	Not such an effective antiseptic as chlorhexidine 4%

Towelling

The anaesthetist will then disconnect the airline and lift the head up so that two towels can be passed under the head and pulled down behind the neck. The top towel is folded over the patient's forehead, or across his face if only the neck needs to be exposed, and secured with a towel clip. The lower towel is now drawn down over the shoulder on both sides, and the chest covered by another towel.

The important point about towelling is to keep in view at all times the edge which will be next to the exposed skin. Consequently, this edge should be held between the two hands and the rest of the towel allowed to trail.

Diathermy

Diathermy is contra-indicated if any explosive agents are used.

Electrical current is frequently used for coagulating blood vessels and cutting through muscles. It can also be used to excise tumour tissue, but biopsy material obtained in this way will be distorted and difficult for the histologist to interpret. The diathermy point carries a positive electric charge which runs to earth through the patient. It is therefore essential to earth the patient by means of a large electrode bandaged to the thigh. Although in children, the pad can be placed under the buttocks, this is inadvisable in adults, because pressure reduces the local blood flow and the tissue may become overheated by the electric current passing through it, leading to a severe burn.

It is essential that no other part of the patient is in contact with a conductor, since the current will often flow through and burn the skin at this point. Before towelling-up, therefore, all theatre staff should ensure that no part of the patient is touching the metal fittings or the metal table top.

Assisting at operations

To assist well requires an informed knowledge of the steps in the operation, concentration and stamina.

Many surgical instruments, for example artery forceps and some suture holders, have a ratchet device to keep them closed. The assistant must be adept at opening and closing these with either hand.

Scissors inexpertly wielded can be a danger both to the patient and the surgeon. Scissors can be most accurately controlled if the thumb and ring finger are placed in the rings and the tip of the index finger placed along the shaft. Ligatures or sutures should be cut with the *ends* of the blades; scissors seldom need be opened more than 1 cm at the tip and the blades should be held at right angles to the skin.

If swabbing, take care not to re-introduce into the mouth (and hence the larynx!) any roots, teeth, etc, that may have been placed on the swab with the intention of disposing of them.

Biopsy specimens

The houseman is responsible for sending the biopsy, with the correct form duly filled in, to the laboratory (see Section 1.5 for biopsy technique).

If a frozen section biopsy is to be taken at operation, the houseman should write out the request form *before* scrubbing-up, and check with the laboratory by telephone to ensure that they will be ready to process the specimen.

Ensure that the necessary specimens are collected. For example, if immunological tests are required (direct immunofluorescence), the tissue must be snap-frozen, while if tuberculosis is suspected, some of the tissue should be sent unfixed, for culture.

Operation records

In ink (usually red), record in the case notes:

(a) the name of the operator and assistant;
(b) the name of the anaesthetist;
(c) the name of the nurse;
(d) date, time and place of operation;
(e) the overall description of the operation and, especially, any deviations from routine or any complications;
(f) any blood loss;
(g) post-operative instructions.

Note: Remember possible medicolegal implications.

7.7 Care of post-operative complications (Tables 7.4 to 7.6)

General post-operative care

The early post-operative period is one of the most dangerous times for the patient, who is recovering from an anaesthetic and who has impaired reflexes. It is imperative to ensure that the airway is protected until the patient recovers his reflexes. The patient *must* be kept in the tonsillar or head injury position (Chapter 8) with an airway in place and *constantly* attended by a trained person, until his reflexes have recovered.

If the patient is slow to regain consciousness, *call the anaesthetist* and carry out the following checks:

(1) airway and respiration;
(2) pulse and BP;
(3) pupil diameter and reactivity;
(4) consider whether there has been a myocardial infarct or other medical complication.

About 50% of patients have some complaint after GA, particularly transient and self-resolving drowsiness, hangover, nausea, sore throat (after intubation and/or packing), aches or pains (from suxamethonium). Prescribe, for use as required, an analgesic and anti-emetic. *Remember to give any medication the patient should normally receive daily* (eg anticonvulsants). Monitor the temperature, pulse, respiration and blood pressure (Figure 7.1).

Post-operative oral complications and care

Complications may affect the mouth or other areas.

Wound pain
In the first 24 hours post-operatively, wound pain should be controlled with analgesics (Section 5.5) given regularly. Post-operative wound pain is usually present for the first few days after operation; at first it is constant, but eventually is present only on moving. If it persists longer than this, or increases, it is likely that there is some pathological process, such as a wound infection, present (eg dry socket).

Severe pain may need to be controlled by morphine or Omnopon given subcutaneously every 4–6 hours. The dosage and drug used will depend on the weight and the age of the patient. For a small adult, 10 mg morphine will usually suffice. For the heavier adult, 15 mg morphine or 20 mg Omnopon may be needed.

The effect of opiates is often more pronounced in the elderly, where they

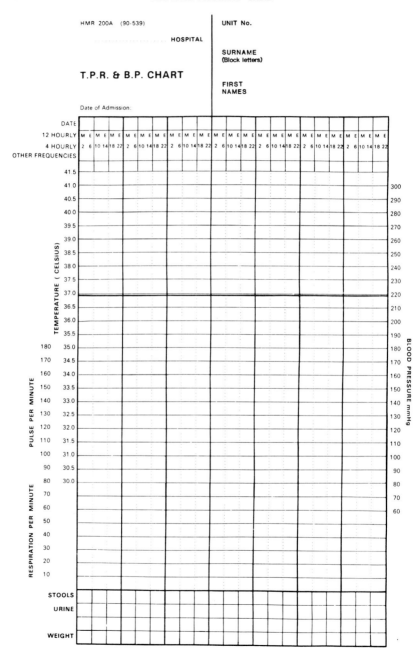

Fig. 7.1 Temperature, pulse, respiration and blood pressure chart.

should be used with great caution. Opiates can cause respiratory depression and are contra-indicated in patients with a head injury.

Wound infection (see also Section 5.7)
In most cases, the diagnosis of infection is obvious since, at about 4 to 8 days after operation, the patient is pyrexial, the wound is inflamed, swollen and tender, and there may be a discharge of pus, and pyrexia.

If pus is draining, there may be no need to give antibiotics, as the infection may settle within a few days. However, pus or a swab should be taken to identify the organism and test sensitivity to antibiotics. If the wound is not draining but is fluctuant, one or more stitches should be removed from the most inflamed area, sinus forceps inserted and gently opened. If the wound infection is only trivial, with no obvious suppuration, antibiotics alone may suffice. Infection under neck flaps is particularly dangerous as the carotid artery may be eroded and burst, which is usually lethal.

Dry socket
Diagnosis is usually obvious. The patient complains of increasing and sometimes severe pain 2–4 days after extraction, often with halitosis and an unpleasant taste. The socket is empty of clot, but may contain debris. The affected area is very tender to palpation.

Radiography is usually needed to exclude retained roots, foreign body, fracture or other pathology. If there are additional features such as pyrexia, intense pain or neurological changes (eg labial anaesthesia), the possibility of acute osteomyelitis or a fracture must be considered.

The principles of treatment of dry socket are:

(1) Gentle irrigation of the socket with warm (50°C) normal saline or aqueous 0·2% chlorhexidine.
(2) Gently dress the affected socket to permit granulation. A number of different concoctions may be used, suggesting that there is little significant difference in efficacy between them.
(3) Analgesics (Section 5.5).

Oedema
The amount of oedema that occurs post-operatively varies between individual patients, but can be reduced by minimising:

- the duration of operation;
- the trauma, in terms of lifting of the periosteum and removal of cortical bone.

Some operators use corticosteroids (Section 5.8), ice packs or other methods to reduce oedema.

Trismus

Trismus can be reduced by minimising the same factors as for oedema, and also by minimising the stripping of muscle off bone.

Young patients in general respond best to operation and there may therefore be sense in, for example, early removal of third molars.

Antral complications

In case of loss of a tooth or root into the antrum, radiograph the area (periapical, occlusal ±OM) to locate the object. If it is extra-mucosal, remove with a sucker or other instrument and use primary closure. If not, further operation will be required. In the meantime, give antimicrobial and nasal decongestant. In the case of an oro-antral fistula (OAF), primary closure may be possible if this is detected early. Other OAFs may close spontaneously, or may need flap closure. Patients should not blow their nose. Give antimicrobial and nasal decongestant (Table 5.3).

Post-operative non-oral complications and care

Deep vein thrombosis (Table 7.6)

The consequences of deep vein thrombosis (DVT; phlebothrombosis) can include:

- local pain and swelling (of the calf usually);
- pulmonary embolism (may be lethal);
- late development of varicose veins, etc.

Predisposing causes include:

- major operation with immobility of legs;
- elderly;
- obese;
- pregnancy or the contraceptive pill.

Prophylaxis. This is indicated in those with a history of DVT, the elderly and the obese, if likely to be immobilised after operation.

Most methods are of unproven value, except low dose subcutaneous heparin (5000 units 2 hours pre-operatively and then 8–12-hourly for 5 days post-operatively), with leggings for intermittent pressure. An alternative is aspirin 300 mg orally, 3 times a day, plus dipyridamole 100 mg orally 3 times a day from 2 days pre-operatively to 5 days post-operatively.

Diagnosis
(*a*) Clinical: leg tender, warm, oedematous.
(*b*) Investigations: venography; Doppler ultrasound; radio-iodine fibrinogen uptake.

Management
- Bed rest until pain and oedema resolve
- Leg exercises.
- Leg bandaging.
- Anticoagulation (or streptokinase). IV heparin for 4–10 days depending on severity of DVT; then warfarin for at least 3 months
- Avoid oestrogen (eg contraceptive pill).
- If pulmonary embolism is suspected (dyspnoea; chest pain):
    (1) Consult the physicians.
    (2) Give 100% oxygen.
    (3) Give pethidine 50 to 100 mg IV or diamorphine 5 mg IV

Post-operative jaundice
Liver disease
Halothane hepatitis may occur if there are repeated administrations.
Gilbert's syndrome: a benign disorder in which jaundice may follow anaesthesia, ingestion of alcohol, or starvation.
Viral hepatitis (uncommon, may follow blood transfusion).
Sepsis (rare).
Drugs: erythromycin *estolate*.

Others
Haemolysis (rare – in haemolytic anaemias or incompatible transfusion).
Resorption of blood from haematoma (rare).
Incidental disease (gallstone disease).

Problems with eating
Apart from nausea and dysphagia and possibly transient anorexia, some patients, especially those with intermaxillary fixation, may need a special soft or liquidised diet. Consult the dietician.

Special diets may also be required for other reasons including:
- Religious grounds.
- Ethical grounds (vegetarians and vegans).
- Diabetes mellitus.
- Those on MAOI.
- Severe liver or renal disease.

Table 7.4 Immediate post-operative complications

System	Complication	Comments	Post-op observations required
Cardiovascular	Haemorrhage	See Table 7.8 and Section 8.2	Haemoglobin, BP, pulse rate
	Hypotension	Usually caused by autonomic suppression from GA Treat by placing patient head down and giving vasopressor IV (ephedrine 5–15 mg or metaraminol 0·5–5 mg)	BP, pulse rate
	Cardiac arrest	See Section 4.6	Conscious level BP, pulse rate
Respiratory	Obstruction	Place patient in 'tonsillar' position post-operatively. Snoring or stridor suggest obstruction Treat by extending head, using pharyngeal airway (eg Guedel airway) and aspirating with sucker. Chest radiograph to exclude aspirated foreign body if recovery impaired (see Section 4.1)	Respiratory rate
	Depression	Often caused by drugs. Suggested by shallow or slow breathing and cyanosis Treat by ventilating with oxygen and giving naloxone 0·4 mg or doxapram 2 mg IM or IV. Maintain airway	
Gastro-intestinal	Nausea, vomiting	May be caused by drugs or swallowed blood. Protect airway and give metoclopramide 5 mg IM or 10 mg orally; or domperidone orally 10 mg for teenagers (or see anti-emetics in Table 7.2). If there is inhalation of any vomit, suck out the pharynx and larynx. Give hydrocortisone 200 mg IV and call the physician, to avoid possible bronchospasm, pulmonary oedema and circulatory collapse (Mendelson's syndrome). Aminophylline and antimicrobials may be indicated.	

Patients with difficulty eating should be weighed daily. Nutrition may need to be given:

(a) by nasogastric or orogastric tube: continuous infusion of a liquid feed is now preferred, since intermittent feeding may cause diarrhoea.

Table 7.5 Post-operative complications appearing usually within first 24 hours

System	Complication	Comments
Pharynx	Sore throat	Endotracheal intubation or throat pack may be responsible. Gargle with soluble aspirin
Neuromuscular	Muscle pains	Suxamethonium frequently causes pain in the back and shoulders
	Nerve damage	Pressure, or extravenous extravasation of drugs may be responsible
Respiratory[a]	Infection, atelectasis	Atelectasis and infection are predominantly problems in smokers or those with pre-existent respiratory disease. Exclude aspiration of foreign body. Consider antimicrobials and physiotherapy
Cardiovascular	Superficial venous thrombosis	Superficial vein thrombosis may be caused by diazepam, propanidid, dextrose, or thiopentone
Renal	Urinary retention	Usually functional. Sit patient up. Give analgesia if abdominal pain. Give warm bath. If all else fails, catheterise or give carbachol
Central nervous system	Confusion or collapse	May be due to one of several factors: Over-sedation or drug reaction Pain Respiratory failure or infection Myocardial infarction Urinary retention or infection Dehydration Metabolic disturbance (eg diabetes) Septicaemia Stroke or other CNS disorder

[a]May take up to 72 hours to appear.

(b) parenterally, ie via an IV catheter in the subclavian or jugular veins. Total parenteral nutrition (TPN) is now fairly commonplace. In addition to weighing regularly, it is necessary to monitor fluid balance, blood glucose, urea and electrolytes, and liver function.

7.8 Shock

Shock is defined as the syndrome of:
- Hypotension.
- Acidosis.
- Oliguria (urine output less than 400 ml/24 hours for the average adult).

Causes include:
- Hypovolaemia (loss of blood or body fluids).

Table 7.6 Post-operative pyrexia

Usual time of appearance (days)	Causes	Prevention	Management
0–3	Septicaemia	Aseptic techniques especially with intravenous infusions	Antimicrobials
	Transfusion reaction	See Section 7.10	Stop transfusion, ± chlorpheniramine 4 mg orally 4 times daily
	Drug reactions, eg to halothane	Avoid repeated exposure	Obtain medical advice[a]
1–3	Respiratory complications Infection Bronchopulmonary segmental collapse	Stop patient smoking Physiotherapy Antimicrobials Avoid respiratory depressants	Drainage (physiotherapy) Antimicrobials ± oxygen Aspiration of obstruction
3–5	Localised infection	Aseptic technique Minimal trauma Antimicrobials	Drainage Antimicrobials
6–10	Deep vein thrombosis/ pulmonary embolism (see Section 7.7)	Avoid pressure on calf Low dose heparin 5000 units SC 2 hours before and every 8–12 hours after surgery	Rest Bandage Anticoagulants ± streptokinase 250 000–600 000 units IV over 30 minutes, then 100 000 units hourly

[a] This may be malignant hyperpyrexia.

- Bacteraemia.
- Acute respiratory obstruction.
- Vascular obstruction.
- Cardiac failure.
- Adrenocortical insufficiency.
- Neurogenic.
- Allergic.

Management
If untreated, shock may lead to cerebral hypoxia, acute renal failure and death.

(1) Lay patient flat with legs raised.
(2) Maintain airway; give oxygen.
(3) Set up a central venous pressure line (see below).
(4) Monitor pulse and blood pressure.
(5) Catheterise (12F gauge Foley catheter) to monitor urine output hourly.
(6) Treat manifestations (Table 7.7).
(7) Establish and, where possible, treat the cause; consult a physician.

Plasma volume expanders (Table 7.8)
These are useful as a temporary measure for replacing the volume lost in acute haemorrhage, while blood is being grouped and cross-matched.

Crystalloids (eg saline) are not satisfactory for this purpose as they do not remain intravascularly. Gelatins, dextrans, hydroxyethyl starch or plasma protein fraction should be used. However, the latter carries the risk that it may transmit viral infections.

Substantially salt-free freeze-dried preparations of albumins are available, which can be reconstituted with distilled water to give the required protein concentration.

Table 7.7   Treatment of shock

Manifestation	Management
Hypotension	IV Infusion. Monitor CVP
Acidosis	IV sodium bicarbonate 8·4% (about 200 MEq/24 hours)
Oliguria	IV infusions as above. Plus diuretic, eg IV mannitol 100 ml of 25% solution
Hypoxia	Give oxygen
Capillary sludging	Give low molecular weight dextran IV (dextran 40 in glucose 5%; Lomodex 40 or Rheomacrodex)

Table 7.8 Plasma volume replacement

Product	Used in	Comments
Gelatins	Severe acute haemorrhage (before blood available)	Lack the osmotic diuresis of dextrans, but have their other disadvantages Give IV infusions (Gelofusine or Haemacel)
Dextrans	Severe acute haemorrhage (before blood available) Severe burns	Take blood for grouping and cross-matching before starting dextrans as they interfere with these procedures. They only replace volume, not oxygen-carrying capacity. May be dangerous in congestive cardiac failure, renal failure and coagulopathies Dextran 70 (Lomodex 70, Macrodex) is the only dextran really suitable. Others are either large (110, 150) and cause red cell aggregation or small (40) and do not remain in the circulation
Hydroxyethyl-starch	Severe acute haemorrhage	May interfere with blood clotting

Table 7.9 Approximate ionic contents of fluids

One bottle replacement fluid	Na^+	K^+	Cl^-	HCO_3^- or equivalent	H^+ or equivalent	Calories/litre
Sodium chloride (150 mmol/litre (isotonic saline)	150	0	150	0	0	0
Glucose 5% (dextrose)	0	0	0	0	0	200
Sodium chloride 30 mmol/litre with 4·3% glucose	30	0	30	0	0	170
Sodium lactate 160 mmol/litre	160	0	0	160	0	0
Sodium bicarbonate 150 mmol/litre	160	0	0	160	0	0

Central venous pressure measurement

Central venous pressure (CVP) measurement assesses pressure in the region of the right atrium and is a useful guide to fluid replacement in shocked, ill and hypovolaemic patients. Setting up a CVP line is a procedure requiring skill and is associated with potential dangers outside the scope of normal activities of junior dental surgeons. The causes of change in CVP include those listed in Table 7.10.

7.9 Intravenous infusions (Table 7.7)

Intravenous (IV) infusions are used to:

- Replace blood volume.
- Give fluids parenterally.
- Feed patients parenterally.
- Correct some anaemias.

Fluid can be lost to the body by several routes and, depending on the quantity and the particular fluid lost (Table 7.11) can lead to:

- Circulatory failure.
- Disturbed electrolyte balances (Table 7.11).

Table 7.10   Changes in central venous pressure

Falling	Rising

(1) Loss of blood volume
     Bleeding
     Dehydration
	(1) Circulatory overload
	     Overtransfusion

(2) Impaired venous return	(2) Cardiac failure

(3) Increased cardiac efficiency	(3) Raised intrathoracic pressure
	     Haemothorax
	     Pneumothorax
	     Pleural effusion
	     Cardiac tamponade

Table 7.11   Electrolyte losses

Body fluid	Electrolyte concentrations (mmol/litre)			Fluid lost in
	Na^+	K^+	Cl^-	
Serum	135–140	3·5–5·0	98–106	Burns Peritonitis
Gastric	60	9·5	100	Vomiting
Biliary	145	5·5	100	Vomiting
Pancreatic	140	5·0	75	Diarrhoea
Small intestinal	120	5·0	100	Fistulae

Post-operatively, fluid and electrolyte disturbances may also appear because of:

- Blood loss during operation.
- Retention of sodium and loss of potassium as a reaction to trauma (this response persists for at least 24 hours).
- Inadequate fluid intake orally.
- Losses of body fluids.

Children, in particular, are prone to dehydration.

Assessment of sodium and water balance is based on:

- History and clinical examination.
- Daily fluid balance chart (fluid intake and loss, including urine output).
- Daily body weight.
- Plasma urea and electrolytes (hyponatraemia is commonly due to water excess, rather than sodium depletion).
- Haemoglobin and PCV.

Dehydration causes thirst at an early stage, but clinical signs appear only when 3 litres or more of fluid have been lost in an adult. Features include:

- Reduced urine output (normal is in excess of 50 ml/hour).
- Dry mouth and conjunctivae.
- Diminished skin elasticity.
- Cold extremities, pallor.
- Increasing pulse rate with a slow fall in blood pressure.
- Plasma urea level increases.
- Haemoglobin and PCV rise (unless there is haemorrhage).

Fluid replacement therapy is based on:

- Supplying the normal intake of fluids and electrolytes (water, 30 ml/kg/24 hours; Na^+ 1·4 mmol/kg/24 hours; K^+ 1·0 mmol/kg/24 hours, for adults).
- Replacing additional losses from the specific clinical situation.
- Modifying the above requirements where renal function is impaired.

The following IV solutions are roughly isotonic and are used specifically to supply:

Water: 5% dextrose (glucose)
Sodium: 0·9% sodium chloride (150 mmol/litre)
Sodium and bicarbonate: 1·4% sodium bicarbonate (150 mmol/litre).

Potassium must only be given with great caution, as it can interfere with cardiac function. Potassium (usually as potassium chloride) can be added to the above solutions, or solutions are available to which potassium in different concentrations has already been added. The maximum concentration of potassium to be given in infused fluid is 40 mmol/litre. The maximum rate of infusion = 13 mmol (1 g)/2 hours.

Post-operative fluid balance in an adult can usually be maintained, providing there are no losses of body fluids (eg through vomiting) by infusing as in Table 7.12. However, fluid balance should always be assessed carefully.

Drip rate:

$$\text{Drops per min} = \frac{\text{Drops in 1 ml} \times \text{Total volume to be given (ml)}}{\text{Total infusion time (min)}}$$

Setting up an intravenous infusion

Asepsis
When indwelling intravenous cannulae are to be used, the operator's hands and nails must be thoroughly washed. Wear gloves and a mask and use strict asepsis; introduction of bacteria may result in bacteraemia or suppurative thrombophlebitis, with serious consequences.

Equipment
Most intravenous cannulae now consist of an outer, non-irritant plastic cannula with a central needle. In general, the largest possible cannula should be used, to ensure an adequate flow.

Intravenous giving sets are available as disposable units of two types. The first, for blood and blood products, has an upper chamber containing plastic gauze to remove any clot and a lower chamber containing a plastic ball valve. Blood can therefore be pumped, using the hand, from this lower chamber into the patient by virtue of the ball valve. The second type of giving set, for non-sanguinous solutions, has a single chamber only.

Find out how the system works *before* inserting the cannula. You will need:

Table 7.12   Rough guide to post-operative fluid balance

Post-operative day	5% dextrose (litres)	Isotonic saline (0·9% sodium chloride) (litres)
1	2	–
2	3	1

(1) A bottle of sterile normal saline and an intravenous giving set, ready filled, with airlocks removed. Even though the 'drip' might be required for giving other fluids, start with saline, since any accidents in setting up the 'drip' will not result in the wastage or spillage of other fluids.

(2) Intravenous cannulae (have at least two available). These must be of a gauge appropriate to deliver the fluid at the required rate. Blood transfusion necessitates gauge 14 and most fluids at least gauge 16–18.

(3) Sterile swabs, antiseptic solution, forceps, tourniquet or sphygmomanometer.

(4) Adhesive tape cut into at least four strips of good length, bandages or netting, and a splint.

(5) Syringes, needles and local anaesthetic solution.

(6) Syringe and specimen tubes for blood sampling.

The use of two- or three-way taps or of burette type infusion sets, and any situation where drugs are frequently added to the infusion apparatus, are particularly liable to result in infection.

Sites
A straight vein away from a joint is best.

The forearm veins. The cephalic vein at the level of the radial styloid which, when the forearm is pronated and the hand pulled into ulnar deviation, is very suitable for cannulation. Splintage is not usually necessary and the patient can therefore move the arm freely.

The antecubital fossa. This is the easiest site for insertion of cannulae, but, because splintage is required, mobility of the arm is reduced.

Veins of the dorsum of the hand. These are useful, since mobility of the limb is retained, but the veins are small and venepuncture is painful. Avoid if drugs, irritant solutions such as dextrose, or large volumes are to be given.

Avoid veins of the lower limb, since there is a risk of thrombophlebitis and of deep vein thrombosis. Only use these in cardiac arrest or for parenteral feeding.

Procedure (fig. 7.2)
(If a 'renal' patient is involved, ask the Renal Unit to carry out the procedure, since the veins are very precious.)

(1) Cleanse the skin.

(2) *Local anaesthesia.* If the patient is nervous or the cannula large, give

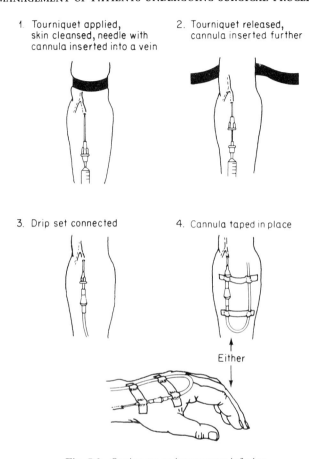

1. Tourniquet applied,
skin cleansed, needle with
cannula inserted into a vein

2. Tourniquet released,
cannula inserted further

3. Drip set connected

4. Cannula taped in place

Either

Fig. 7.2   Setting up an intravenous infusion.

0·5–1% lignocaine without adrenaline 0·2–0·5 ml intradermally over the cannulation site.

(3) *Insertion of cannula.* Essentially the same as insertion of a needle for venepuncture. The needle and cannula are usually attached to the syringe for convenience. Insert the needle obliquely through the skin and enter the vein; blood will be seen tracking up the cannula. Without inserting the needle further, push the plastic outer cannula gently into the vein, remove the needle, take a blood sample for storage of serum in case blood transfusion becomes needed, and then attach the cannula attached to the giving set containing sterile 0·9% saline (but see p. 216). Begin the IV infusion; if the cannula has been inserted correctly and

the tourniquet removed, the flow should be even and rapid. Adjust the rate of infusion as required. Fix the cannula and 'drip' set tubing with the tape. If the cannula has been placed in the antecubital fossa, a splint is required to keep the elbow extended, because otherwise the cannula may kink or pierce the vein.

(4) *Checking of infusion fluids.* Inspect clear fluids for haziness or turbidity in a good light against a dark background, while the container is inverted and gently shaken. A slight swirl of contaminating material may be seen at this time, but will be undetectable once the container has been shaken. If the fluid is not crystal clear and free from particles, it should not be used. The supernatant plasma of blood bottles should show no haemolysis or fibrin web.

The clear fluids include water used to reconstitute dried plasma as well as solutions of dextrose, sodium chloride, etc (see Table 7.9). When satisfied with the fluid, change the saline drip.

(5) *Changing of equipment and cannulae.* Change equipment connected to an IV cannula every 48 hours. When giving a slow infusion over a prolonged period, use a small needle and change every 24–48 hours to a new site. Change dressings as often as necessary to keep the site dry.

(6) Injections into giving sets should be reduced to a minimum. Check that what you are injecting is compatible with the solution in the infusion set. Before injecting into the tubing, clean the injection site with chlorhexidine in 70% spirit and allow to dry.

(7) Rapid infusion of intravenous fluids may be required to maintain life. The first essential is that a large cannula is inserted into a large vein (doubling the size of the cannula will increase the flow rate 16 times; increasing the head of pressure to four times normal will only double the flow rate). Blood or fluid may be given rapidly either by squeezing or pumping the *lower* chamber of a blood transfusion giving set, or by the use of a Martin's pump. The drip set tubing is threaded through the rollers of the pump and the handle rotated to increase the rate of fluid replacement. If large amounts of stored blood are to be given rapidly, the temperature of the blood should be raised by first circulating the blood through a blood warmer (a length of intravenous tubing placed in a bath of pre-warmed fluid at 37°C).

Fifty millilitres of sodium bicarbonate (8·4% solution) should be given for every 3 litres of blood to correct for the acidosis of stored, anticoagulated blood. Ten ml of 10% calcium gluconate intravenously may be necessary to correct for the chelating action of the citrate anticoagulant, but its use is associated with cardiac irregularities and so it should be used with caution. It must always be given slowly with

ECG monitoring. It should not be used where less than 3 litres of blood have been given.

(8) *Monitoring.* Check urea and electrolytes daily (Tables 7.11 and 7.13).

Complications

Difficulty with setting up IV infusions

Obese patients. As with venepuncture, you need patience, palpation and correct pressure. Very often the site of a previous successful venepuncture gives a clue.

Hypotensive patients. The sphygmomanometer is most useful. Allow adequate time for the veins to fill and use good lighting. Palpate the veins prior to cannulation.

The patient with 'no veins'. Although unlikely to occur, you may feel that this is the case with some patients. When a suitable vein cannot be found:

(1) Go systematically through the sites of venepuncture both looking and feeling. Use a sphygmomanometer.
(2) Ask a colleague to help.
(3) In an emergency, an ordinary 20-gauge needle may be inserted into a small vein and enough fluid pumped through this to maintain life, or ask for help to do a cut-down on other sites, such as the saphenous, jugular or subclavian veins.

'Drip' failure

On initial inspection you may see that the drip is not working, but that the arm is swollen and tender. In this event, the cannula has probably pierced

Table 7.13 Average water and salt balance in healthy adults per 24 hours

		Water (ml)		Sodium (mmol)
Intake[a]	Moist food and drink	2 000	Food, drink, seasoning	170
	Dry food and oxidation	500		
Pool	Plasma	3 000	Plasma	450
	Tissue fluid	12 000	Rest of body	3 500
	Cell fluid	30 000		
Output	Insensible loss	1 000	Insensible loss	–
	Urine	1 300	Urine	150
	Faeces	200	Faeces	20
	Sweat	Variable	Sweat	Variable

[a]Minimum requirement: water 1500 ml; 50 mmol sodium. Normal intake of potassium is 80 mmol/24 hours.

the vein and fluid has infused into the subcutaneous tissues. Remove such a 'tissued' drip and, if IV fluids are still required, put another up in another site. If the arm is inflamed, send the cannula tip for bacteriological examination.

If the drip has not 'tissued':

(1) Check that the drip has been fully opened and that there is nothing constricting the arm (eg the sphygmomanometer cuff).
(2) Inspect the site. If it is inflamed, is the vein tender, or is thrombophlebitis present? In either case, take the drip down immediately. Again, send the cannula tip for culture.
(3) If the site is not inflamed, it is likely that the vein has clotted or is in spasm. If the clot is recent, it may be dislodged by gentle pressure from a syringe containing either *sterile* saline or citrate solution. Use even and firm pressure and a small quantity of fluid (less than 10 ml), because of the danger of embolism. The use of low dose heparin (50 units of Hepsal *or* 200 units of Hep-Flush) injected every 6 hours will reduce drip failure without producing identifiable anticoagulation, but should be avoided if there is a bleeding tendency.
(4) If the drip is just going slowly, flush out the cannula with citrate solution or raise the bottle of intravenous fluid as high as possible.

Superficial thrombophlebitis
Mostly caused by chemical irritation, phlebitis presents with local pain, swelling and erythema. Remove the cannula and apply warm packs to the area.

Fever
When a patient receiving IV fluids develops a pyrexia for no apparent reason, the intravenous apparatus should be considered as a possible source of infection. Take a blood culture and a bacteriological swab from the injection site. Send bottle, drip set and cannula to the laboratory in a polythene bag, plus any recently used containers of intravenous fluids or containers of drugs which have been injected. If the patient is seriously ill, or if it is suspected that the fluid in the container may be contaminated, inform a consultant microbiologist urgently.

Septicaemia may develop in patients receiving intravenous therapy. Although uncommon, its consequences may be serious and even fatal. Bacteria may be introduced by intravenous infusion in several ways:

• Contamination before use (rare).

- Contamination during the setting up of the infusion, or during the course of the infusion, despite filtration of the entering air.
- Injection of infected material into drip. Some Gram-negative bacilli grow rapidly in solutions at room temperature. Do not use multidose containers more than once if for IV use.
- Infection may occur where the cannula enters the skin, especially if this area remains moist or if the cannula is not inserted aseptically.
- The cannula may cause venous thrombosis, which may become infected and a source of septic emboli.

Embolisation of catheter material
Take great care not to divide the cannula and produce an embolus.

Circulatory overload
The infusion of fluids too quickly or in large quantities, particularly to elderly patients or those with cardiac failure, may cause circulatory overload. This is potentially dangerous since it may precipitate congestive cardiac failure with pulmonary oedema (persistent cough, frothy sometimes pink blood-stained sputum, dyspnoea). The neck veins are distended and chest examination reveals rales (crepitations).

Avoid this by infusing slowly (using a CVP line in ill patients), using packed red cells rather than whole blood, and giving a diuretic. Manage the overload by stopping the infusion, giving a diuretic such as frusemide 20–40 mg IV, plus subcutaneous morphine 15 mg plus atropine 1 mg, and administering oxygen.

7.10 Transfusion of blood and blood products

Indications
Loss of less than 10% of blood volume may well be compensated, but losses of 20%, or haemoglobin dropping below 9 g/dl or more, require replacement by blood transfusion. Failure to transfuse may lead to persistent hypotension, hypovolaemic shock, and acute renal failure.

Blood transfusion can be life-saving, but should only be given when truly necessary, not simply because one is not sure. It carries appreciable risks and should never be undertaken without carefully weighing the possible benefits against the potential hazards, not least those of the transmission of infections (see later).

Dental patients who could need a blood transfusion include:

- Traumatised patients.
- Those with bleeding tendency (eg leukaemia).
- Those who are anaemic pre-operatively.
- Those undergoing surgery with vascular disorder (eg large haemangioma).
- Those undergoing major surgery, particularly around the carotid.

Grouping and cross-matching

Blood must always be grouped and cross-matched before major surgery. Full blood grouping and cross-matching, which is almost always essential, can take up to 3 hours; in an emergency, rapid cross-matching can be done in 20–40 minutes.

The chief danger in blood transfusion is the administration of the wrong blood. This should be minimised by ensuring that specimens for grouping and matching are taken from the correct patient and fully labelled with the patient's first and second names and hospital number, and that the blood to be transfused is carefully checked for the patient's name and number.

Taking the sample and completing the request form

Samples required are 4 ml in a sequestrene (or citrated) tube (Table 1.20), plus 10 ml clotted in a plain tube (Table 1.21). Ideally, the request form for blood transfusion and the details on the blood specimen bottle should be completed by the person taking the sample.

Correct identification should be obtained from:

- the patient's name bracelet;
- the patient, if conscious.

Details should never be copied from the request form on to the sample bottle label; when collecting specimens from several patients, it is easy to make a mistake, particularly if there are two patients of the same name, but with slightly different details.

Administering blood or blood products to the patient (Table 7.14)

Packed red cells are preferred for non-acute transfusions. On administering blood to the patient, it is important that the final check of identity should be with the patient's wrist bracelet. It is occasionally necessary to remove a patient's identity bracelet, for example, in the operating theatre to gain access to the veins in the wrist. This is a potentially dangerous situation, as the patient is unconscious and separated from his case notes. It is therefore important that, in such circumstances, the identification label should be removed from the old bracelet, put in a new one, and attached to the patient

Table 7.14   Blood and blood products[a]

Product	Used in	Comments
Whole blood	Acute blood loss of more than 1 litre	With massive transfusions there may be citrate-induced bleeding tendency or citrate intoxication. Stored blood may cause hyperkalaemia and has relatively few platelets. Whole blood may cause circulatory overload
Autologous blood	Elective surgery	Avoids cross-infection
Packed red cells	All non-acute transfusions	Less likely than whole blood to cause circulatory overload. More economic since plasma is saved for other uses
Platelet concentrates	Bleeding tendency caused by thrombocytopenia or platelet dysfunction (including leukaemia)	Limited shelf-life (3–5 days depending on storage conditions). Do not administer without consulting haematologists
Leukocyte-poor blood	To restrict leukocyte sensitisation	Used mainly in aplastic anaemia, thalassaemia, or where there are antibodies from pregnancies or earlier transfusions
Human plasma protein fraction	Severe burns	Unsuitable for use in a bleeding tendency
Fresh frozen plasma	Patients with multiple coagulation defects (eg liver disease)	Contains all clotting factors
Cryoprecipitate	Haemophilia A	Less effective than factor VIII
Factor concentrates	Deficiencies of clotting factors	Use only in treatment of specific clotting defects

[a] There may be low risk of transmitting hepatitis B; non-A, non-B hepatitis; AIDS, etc.

as soon as possible. A second person should also check the blood with the patient's identity.

As a general rule, routine transfusions should be given by day as they can be more constantly observed.

Monitor urine output and blood urea (and fibrin degradation products if using stored blood). See also page 224 regarding citrate and potassium toxicity. Incompatibility reactions may be masked by anaesthesia; therefore, monitor the patient's temperature.

Care of veins

Care of veins, particularly in repeated or prolonged transfusion, is of paramount importance, particularly in renal patients.

Points to remember:

- The most effective single precaution is to ensure that, in high risk situations, infusions are only set up by the most experienced operator available.
- In small or frightened children, a light general anaesthetic will often save trauma to vein, child and operator.
- Dextrose solutions are irritant; do not give these through the same giving set as blood, or sludging and thrombophlebitis will occur.
- A small cannula, preferably a plastic type, is less traumatic than the needle and should be used, particularly for prolonged transfusions.
- Avoid flexures if possible; try to preserve veins and avoid 'cutting down'.

Other points

- Never add *any drug* to blood intended for transfusion. If a drug is to be administered at the same time as blood, give this through a Y-tube inserted into the transfusion apparatus.
- For measures to avoid the risk of infection from intravenous infusions, see Section 7.9.
- One unit of whole blood: (*a*) will raise the haemoglobin by about 1 g/dl and (*b*) contains 200 ml red cells, 250 ml plasma and 63 ml anticoagulant (citrate phosphate dextrose ± adenine).

Complications of transfusion

Minor reactions to transfusion are not uncommon and include pyrexia with urticaria. Manage as follows:

(1) Slow the rate of transfusion.
(2) Administer an antihistamine, eg chlorpheniramine 10 mg IM.
(3) If no improvement within 30 minutes, stop transfusion.

Severe incompatibility reactions include pyrexia, rigors, backache, vomiting, collapse, oliguria and haemoglobinuria, facial flushing, angioedema, hypotension and bronchospasm. Manage as follows:

(1) Stop the transfusion. Ask a physician for advice.
(2) Check the details of the patient with the labels on the blood pack.
(3) Take blood samples from the patient, from a vein away from the infusion site:

(*a*) Two sequestrene samples for grouping and direct Coombs' test, and haemoglobin.

(*b*) Two clotted samples for crossmatching, and incomplete antibodies.

(4) Send the remaining donor blood and any remains of previously transfused blood to the laboratory for:

(*a*) Re-crossmatching.
(*b*) Gram-stain.
(*c*) Culture.

(5) There is no specific treatment, but the patient's blood pressure must be maintained by the use of vasopressor agents and intravenous hydrocortisone. Maintenance of blood volume is of paramount importance and a suitable volume expander should be given until more blood can be cross-matched.

(6) Check urine output, specific gravity and for haemoglobin. Low output or persistent SG below 1·01 indicates renal damage. Consult a physician as a matter of urgency.

Delayed incompatibility reactions

Should jaundice appear on the first to third day following the transfusion, associated with an unexpected fall in the patient's haemoglobin level, inform the laboratory and supply clotted blood samples for detection of antibodies.

Bacterial contamination of blood

- Some bacteria, eg *Escherichia coli*, can survive at refrigerator temperature (4°C). They will multiply at higher temperatures. Therefore, never leave blood packs out of the refrigerator for more than 30 minutes on any occasion before use.
- Never give blood if the plasma is red rather than yellowish, as this implies haemolysis, possibly from infection.
- Never transfuse a damaged pack.
- Accidental transfusion of infected blood is extremely dangerous and causes bacteraemia or septicaemia, with pyrexia, vomiting, diarrhoea, hypotension and sometimes haemorrhages.

Circulatory overload (see Section 7.9)

The danger of this can be reduced by

- Transfusing slowly.
- Transfusing packed red cells rather than whole blood.
- Giving a diuretic, eg frusemide 20–40 mg (Lasix).

Citrate and potassium toxicity

Massive transfusions, particularly to patients with liver disease, may cause citrate toxicity, manifesting with tremors and ECG changes. Avoid by giving a slow injection IV of 10 ml 10% calcium gluconate with every second bottle of blood, in long continuous transfusions (monitor ECG).

Stored blood tends to haemolyse, releasing potassium. A massive transfusion of stored blood may produce hyperkalaemia and can affect cardiac function, even producing cardiac arrest.

Bleeding tendency

Stored blood has low levels of platelets and coagulation factors. Massive transfusions of stored blood (15 units plus) need the addition of platelet concentrates (6 units) and fresh frozen plasma (4 units) to restore haemostatic activity.

When incompatible blood is given during operation, there may be unexplained hypotension or sudden diffuse and spontaneous bleeding. In this event, 500 ml fresh frozen plasma may be of value in replacing missing coagulation factors.

Late complications

See Section 3.8 on AIDS and Section 3.9 on viral forms of hepatitis.

7.11 Discharge of hospital patients and convalescence

Discharge

The patient and relatives should be forewarned as accurately as possible of the date and time of intended discharge. Discharge patients only with the consent of the consultant responsible.

Inform the Admissions Officer and, if transport is needed, also the Ambulance Officer, well in advance of planned discharge, (1 to 2 days at least, where possible). On, or before, the day of discharge, write a discharge letter and give to the patient for delivery to the GDP or send this by post. In some cases it may be necessary to telephone the GDP or GP to brief him on the patient's condition and treatment. Include the following information:

- Date of discharge.
- Operation carried out (and date).
- Subsequent progress.
- Condition on discharge/medications.
- Follow-up treatment required (eg suture removal).
- Date of follow-up appointment.

Arrange for community care, where necessary, with the medical social worker. Also arrange an out-patient follow-up appointment and for the patient to take or collect from the GDP or GP any necessary medication.

Last, but not least, tell the patient what he/she may expect; for example, how long will the swelling persist and what should be done if there are complications or uncertainty.

Convalescence

- Recommendation for convalescence is the responsibility of the consultant in charge of the patient and should be made as early as possible.
- Referrals are usually made in consultation between the Sister and the convalescence secretary or medical social worker.
- The medical information given to the convalescence home secretary must be up-to-date with details of all treatment, and must include particulars of any coexisting disease.
- All drugs must be listed and sent with the patient to the convalescent home.

Irregular discharge

Although it is no part of a dental surgeon's duty to detain patients who are mentally well, against their will, any patient who wishes to take his own discharge against medical advice should have the consequences politely explained to him, in the presence of a witness such as the ward Sister.

Try to contact your immediate senior to see if he can be more persuasive. If you are really concerned because, for example, the patient is postoperative and not in a fit state to discharge himself, speak immediately to the responsible consultant.

If the patient still insists on leaving, ask him to sign a statement accepting responsibility for his own discharge, in the presence of a witness. Record the event in the case notes.

If he takes his own discharge but refuses to sign such a disclaimer, again record the event in the case records, and also ask the witness to sign the case notes, stating that he is 'leaving hospital against medical advice'.

Deaths in hospital

- All deceased patients must be seen by a medically qualified individual in order that the death may be certified.
- Inform your consultant immediately.
- The GP should be notified by a medically qualified person at the same time as the death certificate is completed.

8

The Traumatised Patient

8.1 Maxillofacial trauma: summary of important points

Patients with maxillofacial trauma can be divided into those with:

(1) Fractures of the mandible, who can be readily managed by dental means and who rarely have serious injuries to other parts.
(2) Fractures of the middle or upper third facial skeleton, commonly because of severe trauma (particularly road accidents), who are more likely therefore to have their life threatened because of associated
   (*a*) airway obstruction and/or
   (*b*) head injury and/or
   (*c*) serious trauma to other parts, particularly chest injuries, ruptured viscera, eye injuries, fractures of the cervical or lumbar spine, and fractures of long bones with serious internal bleeding.

Keeping the patient alive is the main priority. Definitive management of maxillofacial fractures, in spite of the frighteningly severe initial disfigurement, comes near the bottom of the list of the patient's priorities. Immediate life-threatening injuries are mainly airway embarrassment, severe bleeding, and intracranial bleeding. Remember:

> **P** Posture
> **A** Airway
> **T** Tongue traction
> **T** Tubes/Tracheotomy
> **E** Examination
> **R** Reassurance of patient
> **N** Notification of specialists, eg neurosurgeons

Finally, remember to keep clear and accurate records, not least because medicolegal proceedings are common.

8.2 Early management of patients with maxillofacial trauma

A   Airway
B   Bleeding, burns
C   Cranium, CNS, CSF, cervical spine, chest
D   Diplopia, dentures, dentition, drugs
E   Eyes, ears
F   Facial lacerations, fractures, foreign bodies
G   Genito-urinary and other injuries, gunshot wounds
H   History
I   Infection

Airway

The single most important consideration in any maxillofacial fracture is preservation of the airway. Cerebral hypoxia will kill a patient within about 3 minutes.

Even with mandibular fractures alone, fragmentation of the anterior part (to which the genial muscles are attached) can allow the tongue to fall back into the airway. The airway can be blocked by blood clot or, rarely, by displacement of a fractured maxilla downwards and backwards towards the pharynx. Teeth, dentures, vomit or foreign bodies may also block the airway.

Removable obstructions must be cleared immediately and the pharynx sucked clear. Backward displacement of the maxilla (very rare) should be reduced by hooking the fingers round the posterior border of the palate and pulling the maxilla forward, steadying the head with the other hand.

Patients with maxillofacial injuries must be placed and transported in the tonsillectomy (head down) position (fig. 8.1). In the conscious or unconscious patient without respiratory problems, the simplest way to maintain a clear airway is by correct positioning, prone or semi-prone, with the foot of the bed elevated. In this position the tongue falls forward and any saliva, blood or gastric content will dribble out rather than be aspirated into the trachea.

An airway placed over the tongue will prevent it falling backwards and occluding the air passages. A nasopharyngeal tube is useful if the lumen can be kept patent. Frequent suction of the mouth and pharynx may be necessary to remove blood, vomit or secretions.

Remember the possibility of damage to the cervical spine; take care not to extend the head.

Stridor may be due to paralysis of the vocal cords or to a plug of mucus or foreign body in the larynx. In any patient with stridor, laryngoscopy should be carried out as an emergency procedure. Laryngeal trauma may result in oedema but this can take up to 12–24 hours to develop.

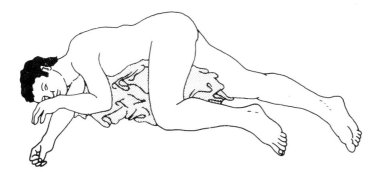

Fig. 8.1   The tonsillar or head injury position.

Laryngoscopy

Stand behind the supine patient, spray the fauces and pharynx with 4% lignocaine and insert the laryngoscope. Check the vocal cords and their movements.

Endotracheal intubation (fig. 8.2)

In patients with acute respiratory obstruction, or in whom cardiac arrest has occurred, this procedure is one of the most important and life-saving. Equipment required includes a Macintosh laryngoscope, Magill forceps and endotracheal tubes (orotracheal and nasotracheal). For females, a number 7 to 9 tube is usually adequate; for males, size 8 to 11 are suitable, depending on the build of the patient. Synthetic plastic tubes are better for long-term use.

(1) If the patient is unconscious, it is usually unnecessary to use muscle relaxants before intubation. If the patient is conscious, give an IV anaesthetic and 50 mg suxamethonium. By resorting to the use of muscle relaxants, an irreversible step has been taken, in that skilled assistance must be available in case it is not possible to pass the endotracheal tube. The houseman therefore must not carry out this procedure on his own.

(2) Stand behind the supine patient.

(3) Remove his dentures.

(4) Insert the laryngoscope and push the tongue to the left. Aspirate mouth and pharynx. Nasotracheal intubation is usually needed for dental procedures; orotracheal intubation is the usual method for emergencies.

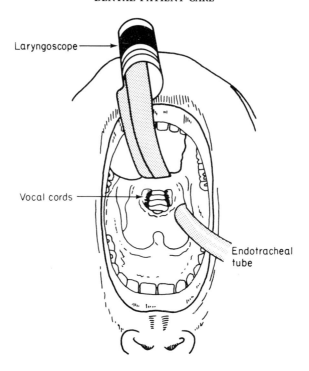

Laryngoscope

Vocal cords

Endotracheal tube

Fig. 8.2   Endotracheal intubation.

(5) Hold the endotracheal tube ready lubricated (with lignocaine gel) in the right hand and with the left hand pull the laryngoscope upwards to expose the epiglottis and vocal cords. As the cords come into view, slip the tube into the trachea using Magill forceps.

(6) Inflate the cuff and connect the tube to an inflation bag. If the tube is properly inserted, the chest should move uniformly with manual ventilation and both lung fields should be auscultated with a stethoscope. The cuff ensures that the trachea is air-tight and prevents aspiration of gastric contents, blood or saliva.

(7) An endotracheal tube should not be left in position for more than about 48 hours. With the newer PVC tubes, this period may be extended slightly, but tracheostomy should be considered if long-term intubation is required.

Laryngostomy (cricothyrotomy)

Indications

Where there is acute laryngeal obstruction or acute respiratory failure but an endotracheal tube cannot be passed, laryngostomy (coniotomy) should be performed as an emergency operation.

Technique

Thrust a wide bore needle (12- to 14-gauge), or cricothyrotome, through the cricothyroid membrane, between the thyroid cartilage and the cricoid cartilage. Connect this needle to a cylinder of oxygen.

This *temporary* procedure must be followed, as soon as possible, by formal tracheostomy and closure of the laryngostomy wound.

Laryngostomy may cause complications (eg laryngitis and laryngeal stenosis) but, if used as a life-saving procedure, these risks are justifiable.

Tracheostomy (tracheotomy)

Indications

See figure 8.3.

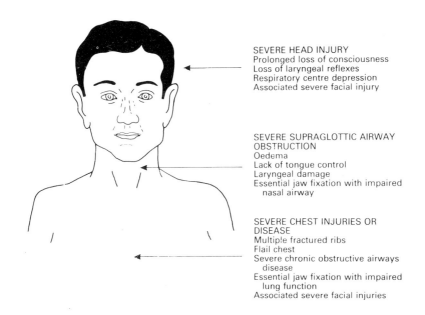

Fig. 8.3 Indications for tracheostomy.

Technique

Tracheostomy should be regarded as an *elective* procedure, normally performed in the operating theatre or intensive care unit, under a general anaesthetic and with an endotracheal tube in position before starting. Tracheostomy is reserved for patients in whom intubation is expected to last for more than 48 hours.

(1) Warn the patient and relatives that he will be unable to speak after the tracheostomy.

(2) Use full sterile precautions and, if possible, operate in theatre.

(3) Tracheostomy tubes may be polyvinyl chloride (PVC) or silver. PVC tubes are less irritant. For the average male, sizes 36 to 39 (French gauge) should be suitable, and for females, sizes 33 to 36. These tubes are cuffed; some have double cuffs to minimise tracheal trauma. Check the connections to the anaesthetic equipment.

(4) Make a transverse incision in the skin of the neck 4–5 cm long, midway between the base of the thyroid cartilage and the suprasternal notch. Divide the tissues down to the deep fascia. Cut the strap muscles vertically in the mid-line and expose the trachea. All bleeding must be stopped before making further incisions.

(5) It is imperative that the first tracheal cartilage is *not* incised or tracheal stenosis will occur. It may not be possible to see tracheal rings 2 to 5 because of overlying thyroid tissue. If this is the case, retract or divide the thyroid isthmus. Clamp either side of the thyroid and divide it to expose the trachea. At this point it is worthwhile comparing the size of the trachea with the proposed tracheostomy tube.

(6) Withdraw the endotracheal tube a little before opening the trachea, so that if difficulties arise, the tube may be replaced rapidly.

(7) Cut out a circular hole in the trachea, after placing artery or tissue forceps on the cartilage so that there is no chance of the portion removed falling into the trachea, or use an inferiorly based flap (Bjork flap), suturing the tracheal cartilage to the skin.

(8) Insert the tracheostomy tube as rapidly as possible. If the patient is anaesthetised and paralysed, there will be no oxygen reaching the lungs during this time and intubation must therefore be carried out with urgency.

(9) Inflate the cuff of the tracheostomy tube and loosely suture the ends of the wound. Knot the tapes of the tube securely at the back of the neck.

(10) The tracheostomy tube itself may then be sutured to the skin with two stitches.

Care of tracheostomy

(1) At least initially, the patient will require frequent tracheal toilet to remove retained secretions. This is a sterile procedure, carried out using masks and gloves. Insert the catheter into the trachea using forceps and apply suction only as the catheter is withdrawn. The catheter is inserted into one main bronchus, then the other. Depending on the clinical state of the patient, suction is repeated as often as required (which may be every 15–30 minutes initially).

(2) Since the cuff of the tracheostomy tube causes pressure on the trachea, it is usual to deflate it for at least a period of 5 minutes every 2 hours. Deflation often induces coughing; therefore, suck out the trachea before and after deflation, and after re-inflation.

(3) Aspirate hourly; send aspirate for culture every 48 hours.

Changing the tracheostomy tube

(1) Cut the tapes securing the tracheostomy tube and remove the dressings.

(2) Using sterile technique, suck out the tracheostomy, deflate the cuff and use suction again.

(3) Gently remove the tube and insert a new one of similar size. A smaller tube must always be available in case the tube cannot be readily re-inserted. Repeat the suction.

The conscious patient and the tracheostomy tube

Some conscious patients with a tracheostomy tube or endotracheal tube rapidly adapt to the situation, even if assisted ventilation is being used. Reassurance and explanation may be all that is required.

However, the presence of the tube in the trachea, together with associated injuries, make some patients restless. Sedation may then be required; phenoperidine 2 mg intravenously may be sufficient, the dose being repeated as required, unless the blood pressure is reduced by the drug. Phenoperidine may also be used in conjunction with droperidol, 5–10 mg IV if extra sedation is required. Diazepam 2–10 mg IV may be used.

Removal of the tracheostomy tube

(1) Remove the tube at the earliest possible moment compatible with the clinical state of the patient, to minimise the dangers of long-term tracheostomy.

(2) As with changing of the tracheostomy tube, have a second, smaller tube available in case there is laryngeal obstruction, or obstruction at the stoma.

(3) Before removing the tube, deflate the cuff for 2–3 days and cover the stoma with a swab.

(4) If the trachea and upper air passages are patent, then the patient should be able to speak and breathe normally. Before removal of the tube, a lateral soft tissue radiograph of the neck is needed, to exclude obstruction higher up in the trachea, for instance an area of granulation tissue above the tube which, on tube removal, will block the tracheal lumen.

(5) Following removal of the tube, which should be done first thing in the morning, observe the patient closely over the next few hours for increasing respiratory difficulty or stridor. If any of these occur, immediately re-intubate.

(6) After successful removal of the tube, it is usually unnecessary to suture the wound; just place a simple dressing.

(7) If the tracheostomy is likely to be required for more than 2–3 days, it is best to change the tube for a silver metal tube, since the inner sleeve can easily be changed to keep the lumen patent. In prolonged tracheostomies, an inner speaking tube can be used.

Complications of tracheostomy
- Bleeding from tracheal ulceration: remove the source of pressure.
- Infection: avoid by using an aseptic technique; treat with antimicrobials.
- Obstruction of tube: deflate cuff and replace tube.

Bleeding
- Severe haemorrhage can lead to cardiac or renal failure or cause fatal cerebral hypoxia.
- Serious bleeding may be concealed, for example into the abdomen from a ruptured viscus (particularly the spleen), or into the thigh from a fractured femur. Haemorrhage into the pleural cavity from fractured ribs can embarrass respiration. Latent haemorrhage can be recognised by:

(*a*) Increasing pulse rate.
(*b*) Falling blood pressure.
(*c*) Increasing pallor.
(*d*) Air hunger.
(*e*) Restlessness.
(*f*) Abdominal rigidity and increasing girth if there is intra-abdominal bleeding.

- Severe nose bleeds that do not cease spontaneously after pressure or after packing with 0·5 inch ribbon gauze, may be controlled with a postnasal gauze pack or by using a Foley balloon catheter passed through the nose into the nasopharynx, softly inflated and then pulled gently back against the posterior nasal choanae.

- Maxillofacial injuries alone, unless associated with a split palate or gunshot wounds, rarely cause severe haemorrhage. A ruptured inferior dental artery usually stops bleeding spontaneously, but bleeding may recur if, for example, there is traction on the mandible. If bleeding recurs, the damaged vessel must be ligated, at open operation if necessary.
- If severe haemorrhage occurs or is suspected:
  - (*a*) Establish an intravenous line (Section 7.9).
  - (*b*) Take blood for grouping and cross-matching.
  - (*c*) Seek a surgical opinion.
  - (*d*) Organise the following quarter-, or half-hourly, observations: pulse rate, blood pressure, respiratory rate, urine output and fluid balance (usually daily).
- Blood transfusion is not needed to replace losses of less than 500 ml in an adult, unless there was pre-existing anaemia, or deterioration of the general condition warrants transfusion (Section 7.10).
- A rising blood pressure and slow pulse, by contrast, indicate a rising intracranial pressure produced by cerebral bleeding or oedema.

Burns
- Burns can be serious injuries and should be treated in Burns or Plastic Surgery Units. Children with burns affecting more than 10% of the body surface area, and adults with over 15% burns, are at special risk because of fluid loss (fig. 8.4).
- First aid treatment of burns includes the following:
  - (1) Ensure adequate airway. Give oxygen if there are respiratory burns or smoke has been inhaled.
  - (2) Cool the area to reduce tissue damage and pain.
  - (3) Superficial (no blisters) or partial thickness (blisters) burns: on the face, leave exposed; on the extremities, dress with silver sulphadiazine cream and enclose in plastic bag.
  - (4) Full thickness burns or those over 15%: call the specialist! Take blood for grouping and cross-matching and put up an intravenous line (Section 7.9). Give 5% dextrose initially. Give analgesia intravenously (morphine 5–15 mg for adults).

Cranium (head injury)
- Head injuries are the main cause of death or permanent disability in patients with maxillofacial injuries.

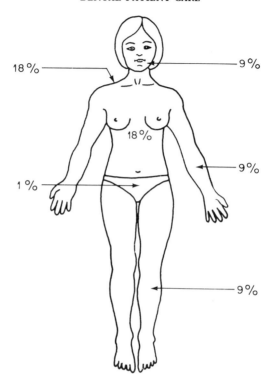

Fig. 8.4 Calculations of the area involved in burns by 'rule of nines'.

- Direct damage to the brain can be the cause of death before the patient reaches hospital, or within the first few days.
- Skull fractures and even mild head injuries can cause epi- or subdural haematomas, causing increased intracranial pressure and possible death.
- The brain is invariably damaged to some degree when consciousness has been lost, even briefly, and sometimes when it has not. Prolonged or increasing loss of consciousness is indicative of serious brain damage (or of other disease interfering with brain function).
- Many patients, even if not comatose, are confused after the injury. Witnesses are needed to give an account of events. Relatives or friends may be able to fill in the patient's medical background.
- Several other complications can contribute to brain damage:
    (*a*) Airway obstruction.
    (*b*) Intracranial haematoma or oedema.

(c) Hypotension.
(d) Meningitis.
(e) Concomitant causes of coma.

It is crucial to establish a baseline level of neurological function and monitor progress with regard to 'neurological observations' using a chart such as in figure 8.5.

Neurological observations
● Conscious level (by far the most important parameter).
● Pupil reaction, pupil size and cranial nerve function (Table 1.15).
● Pulse.
● Blood pressure.
● Respiratory rate and pattern.

Signs and symptoms that suggest development of neurological complications and indicate the urgent need for a neurosurgical opinion
● Deteriorating conscious level.
● Increasing restlessness: behavioural changes.
● Headache.
● Vomiting.
● Focal signs – hemiparesis, dysphasia, focal epilepsy.
● Dilatation of pupil(s).
● Bradycardia.
● Rising blood pressure.

Important examinations
Examination of the head for fractures, scalp wounds (particularly the occipital region) or leakage of cerebrospinal fluid (nose or ears).

Important investigations
● Radiographs (see Table 8.4; see also *Lancet* 1983; **1**: 115).
● Computerised axial tomography (CAT) scan.
● Blood analyses (particularly glucose).
● Urinalysis.

Cerebrospinal fluid leaks
Patients with middle third fractures involving the naso-ethmoidal complex have CSF leaks because of dural tears in about 25% of cases. They are predisposed to develop meningitis, with serious consequences. Dural tears occur also at other sites; CSF may leak either from the nose or into the

Neurological observation chart

		DATE																					
	Frequence of Recordings	TIME																					
Coma Scale	Eyes Open	Spontaneously																					
		To Speech																					
		To pain																					
		None																					
	Best verbal response	Orientated																					
		Confused																					
		Inappropriate Words																					
		Incomprehensible Sounds																					
		None																					
	Best motor response	Obey commands																					
		Localise pain																					
		Flexion to pain																					
		Extension to pain																					
		None																					

Eyes closed by swelling = C

Endotracheal tube or tacheostomy = T

Usually record the best arm response

Blood pressure and pulse rate																					
240																					
230																					
220																					
210																					
200																					
190																					
180																					
170																					
160																					
150																					
140																					
130																					

Temperature (°C)

41
40
39
38
37
36

Pupil size (mm)

○ 1
○ 2
○ 3
○ 4

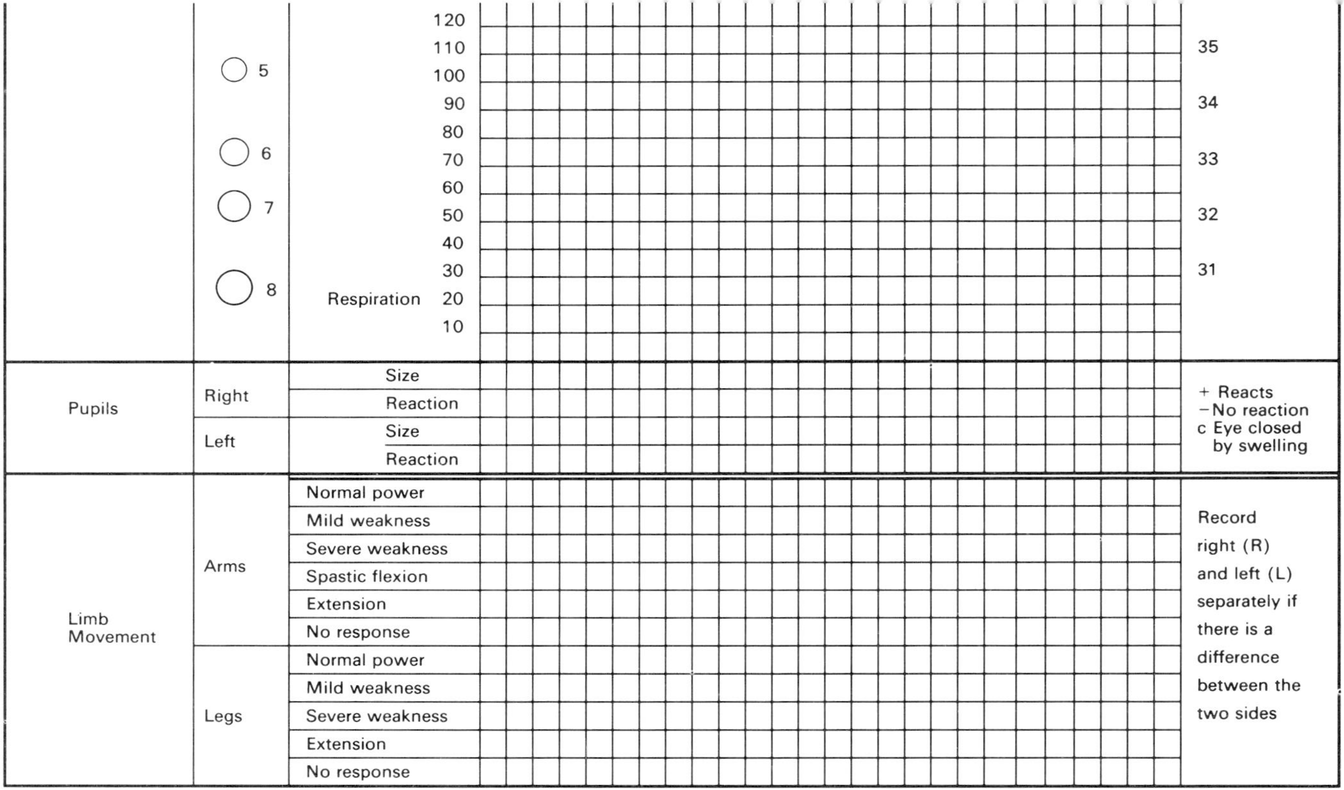

		35	
		34	
		33	
		32	
		31	
		120	
		110	
		100	
		90	
		80	
		70	
		60	
		50	
		40	
		30	
		20	
		10	
		Respiration	
Pupils	Right	Size	+ Reacts
		Reaction	− No reaction
	Left	Size	c Eye closed by swelling
		Reaction	
Limb Movement	Arms	Normal power	Record right (R) and left (L) separately if there is a difference between the two sides
		Mild weakness	
		Severe weakness	
		Spastic flexion	
		Extension	
		No response	
	Legs	Normal power	
		Mild weakness	
		Severe weakness	
		Extension	
		No response	

Pupils scale: 5, 6, 7, 8

Fig. 8.5 Neurological observation chart.

nasopharynx (CSF rhinorrhoea) or from the ear (CSF otorrhoea). CSF leak should be assumed in all high level facial fractures.

CSF is a watery, clear fluid (but is often disguised in the early stages by bleeding). It can be differentiated by its high sugar (use Clinistix) and low protein content (electrophoresis) from serous nasal discharge or lacrimal fluid (which both have a high protein content). If CSF leakage is not seen, but the patient complains of an intermittent salty taste, place him prone, tipped with the face downwards, to provoke an obvious flow of CSF from the nose.

Penicillin is inadequate as prophylaxis against meningitis. The traditional use of sulphadiazine is questionable, because of the many resistant bacteria, particularly *Neisseria meningitidis*. Rifampicin (20 mg/kg) may be preferable, since it reaches the CSF in adequate concentrations and is effective against most of the bacterial causes of post-traumatic meningitis (see Table 8.1).

A neurosurgical opinion is indicated (dural repair may be necessary), particularly when the CSF leak persists for more than 10 days.

Warn the patient not to blow his nose.

Cervical spine injuries

Cervical spine injuries are not infrequent in road traffic accidents. Do not extend the neck until it has been established that the cervical spine is intact,

Table 8.1 Prophylactic antibacterials for patients with compound facial fractures and/or CSF leakages (see also Tables 5.22–5.24)

Drug	Adult dose	Route	Indications
Penicillin	600 mg 6-hourly	IM	Compound facial fracture (for 5–7 days)
Sulphadiazine	500 mg initially IM then 250 mg 6-hourly	IM	
Sulphatriad[b]	4 tabs initially then 2 tabs 6-hourly	O	*One* of these drugs if there is a CSF leakage[a] or compound skull fracture
Sulphadimidine	2 g initially then 1 g 6-hourly	IM or O	
Rifampicin	600 mg daily as single morning dose	O	

[a]Until about 2 days after CSF leakage stops.
[b]Sulphadiazine, sulphathiazole and sulphamerazine.

otherwise you may cause spinal cord damage leading to paralysis or death. Cervical collars applied in the Accident and Emergency Department afford inadequate support if there is a cervical injury, but they do warn of its presence.

Chest injury

If there has been trauma to the chest, careful examination and radiographs are required to exclude fractured ribs, pneumothorax, haemothorax, lung collapse, mediastinal shift, and air under the diaphragm (suggests rupture of an abdominal viscus) or cardiac damage.

If the airway is unobstructed, difficulty in breathing associated with paradoxical movements of the chest and cyanosis may indicate a flail chest. Obtain a medical/surgical opinion, as intermittent positive pressure artificial respiration via an endotracheal tube is then needed.

Diplopia

Diplopia following maxillofacial trauma may be caused by orbital oedema or haemorrhage, displacement of the orbit, or damage to extra-ocular muscles or cranial nerves III, IV or VI. Obtain an ophthalmological surgeon's opinion if there is any suggestion of loss of visual acuity or of diplopia pre- or post-operatively.

Dentures/dentition

Establish the whereabouts of dentures or fragments of dentures and lost teeth or fragments thereof. Any of these may have been lost into the tissues, swallowed or, far more seriously, inhaled (see Sections 4.1 and 4.2). A chest radiograph may be indicated. The management of traumatised teeth is discussed in Section 9.5.

Drugs

Drugs such as alcohol may have been responsible for the trauma. For analgesia avoid opiates, but rather give codeine phosphate 10–20 mg IM. Most patients with compound facial fractures will require antimicrobials (Table 8.1).

Eyes and ears

Obtain an early expert opinion if eye or ear lesions are suspected from the history or examination. Blood in the external auditory meatus may signify a basal skull fracture or, more likely, a condylar fracture. CSF otorrhoea indicates a basal fracture, as may bruising behind the ear.

Facial lacerations

These may cause profuse haemorrhage, which usually appears worse to the patient, relatives and operator than it is. Examine and probe lacerations carefully for foreign bodies such as road dirt, plastic, glass and metal. The repair of facial wounds is not for the beginner and eyelid wounds must always be repaired by the ophthalmic or plastic surgeon. Patients rightly expect the very best cosmetic and functional repair of facial wounds.

Immediate care
(1) Remove relatives, who may be distressed and more upset than the patient.
(2) Facial lacerations can, if necessary, because of other more serious injuries, be left for up to 24 hours for closure, as long as they are dressed with saline packs after haemostasis has been achieved.
(3) Antimicrobials are needed, particularly if lacerations are through and through (usually penicillin; Table 8.1).
(4) Tetanus prophylaxis may be needed (Table 8.2).

Cleaning and debridement of wounds (Table 8.3)
(1) Clean and debride traumatic wounds before closure. Wounds from high velocity missiles should not immediately be closed (see later: Gunshot wounds).
(2) Local analgesia is often sufficient, but consider GA if the wounds may involve foreign bodies, may take more than 30 minutes to repair, involve tissue loss, are difficult to anaesthetise with LA, are large (especially children or females), or involve arterial haemorrhage.

Table 8.2 Prophylaxis against tetanus in the wounded patient

Superficial wound or abrasion		Deep wound, puncture wound or bite	
Immune patient*	Patient not known to be immune	Immune patient*	Patient not known to be immune
Wound debridement; no specific action	Wound debridement; give toxoid[a] (first immunisation)	Wound debridement; give toxoid[a] (booster) unless boosted in previous year ± antibiotics	Wound debridement; penicillin. If seen within 4 hours, give toxoid;[a] if seen later, give anti-tetanus globulin[b]

*Patients who have in the past 5 years been vaccinated or had a booster.
[a]Tetanus toxoid 0·5 ml IM or deep SC.
[b]Anti-tetanus globulin 250 units IM if seen before 4 hours have elapsed; otherwise give 500 units IM.

(3) Clean wounds by washing with a mild antiseptic solution such as aqueous chlorhexidine (0·1%) or hypochlorite. All foreign bodies and dirt should be removed (by scrubbing if necessary). Long-term complications are often caused by failure to remove debris.

(4) Areas suspected of being non-viable by virtue of a bluish colour and diminished capillary return on pressure should be excised until bleeding occurs, along with damaged muscle.

(5) Simple, relatively uncontaminated superficial abrasions should be cleaned with aqueous chlorhexidine 0·1% solution and sterile saline, and dressed with water-rinsable petrolatum gauze and then dry sterile dressings.

(6) Abraded skin contaminated with dirt may heal to cause a tattoo, unless thoroughly cleaned. Such lesions should be vigorously scrubbed clean under anaesthesia, using a soft wire brush and irrigation with 10 volumes per cent hydrogen peroxide.

(7) Do not close lacerations over fractures without first ensuring that the relevant surgeon will not require them as access for exploration.

Wound closure

(1) Consider whether you are the best person to repair the wound.

(2) For most wounds the placement of deep subcutaneous sutures (Table 8.3) to approximate severed layers correctly is the most important part of the procedure. If the deep layers are approximated correctly, the closure of the skin layers is considerably aided, with better function and aesthetics. This is especially important in areas such as the lips and vermilion borders. Resorbable materials such as 3/0 to 4/0 size Dexon, catgut, chromic catgut, or soft gut may be considered (Table 8.3).

(3) Atraumatic needles are generally preferred. For skin sutures usually 3/0 (000·2 metric) black silk or linen or nylon are used, but for facial wounds, 5/0 (1 metric) or 6/0 polypropylene, nylon or silk are preferred (Table 8.3). Monofilament materials are associated with a lower rate of wound infection compared with multifilament sutures. Black silk (3/0) is preferable for oral wounds (pliable and easily seen).

(4) For most oral wounds, insert the sutures approximately 0·5–1 cm apart. Take equal bites of the mucosa so that the edges lie correctly together. Take smaller bites for most facial wounds and insert sutures at more frequent intervals.

(5) Closure of skin wounds by adhesive tapes is convenient, with good cosmetic results and produces a strong wound with little infection. The skin and wound should be thoroughly cleaned as above, and all bleeding within the wound must cease before the tapes are applied. If

Table 8.3 Suture materials in dentistry

Site to be sutured	Suture material	Comments
Intradermal (subcuticular)	6/0 or 5/0 polypropylene or nylon	Stronger than other material; soft; non-irritant
	5/0 or 4/0 polypropylene	Knots easily; simple to remove
Subcutaneous or submucosal	5/0 polyglycolic acid	Absorbable; less irritant than catgut or collagen; stronger than catgut
	5/0 plain or soft catgut	Absorbable
Mucosa	3/0 black silk	Strong but flexible and easily seen
	3/0 plain or soft catgut	Resorbable; useful in children or disturbed patients
	3/0 polyglycolic acid	Resorbable (useful as is gut)

the wound is deep or there is excess fat, then subcutaneous stitches of an absorbable material (Table 8.3) should be inserted first. Only when the wound is completely dry are the tapes (eg Steristrip, Micropore) applied. Avoid tension since otherwise friction blisters may occur.

(6) Tissue adhesives may be valuable in certain cases. Butyl 2-cyano-acrylate is least toxic and can be useful in children.

Care of sutures
Wounds should be cleaned with chlorhexidine 0·1% aqueous solution and Polyfax ointment applied twice daily to prevent scab formation, facilitate suture removal and reduce scarring.

Suture removal
(1) Facial sutures should be removed within 3–5 days, to keep scarring to a minimum; mucosal sutures are removed at 5–7 days.
(2) Remove alternate sutures first to see if wound has healed adequately. If so, remove the remaining sutures a day later. If wounds tends to gape a little, use tapes (not in the mouth).
(3) Many patients are apprehensive and need reassurance.
(4) Clean the wound and surrounding mucosa or skin with aqueous 0·2% chlorhexidine.

(5) Lift the suture with sterile forceps and cut the stitch on one side, as close to the skin or mucosa as possible (this avoids pulling contaminated suture material through the wound).
(6) Pull the suture out using traction on the long end, across the wound so as to avoid pulling apart the edges.
(7) Clean the area again with an antiseptic solution.
(8) With tape-closed wounds, the tapes are left in place for 7–10 days and then gently removed by traction.

Foreign bodies

Common foreign bodies include glass from windscreen lacerations or assaults, plastic from car components, or metal projectile fragments.

(1) Explore wounds with a sterile probe and take relevant soft tissue radiographs. Some glass is radiopaque.
(2) If there is any suggestion of ocular involvement, immediately ask an ophthalmologist to see the patient.
(3) Retain all foreign bodies; they may be of forensic value in subsequent litigation.

Genito-urinary, abdominal, or other injuries

Traumatic injuries, particularly from road traffic accidents or personal violence may well be associated with serious abdominal or other injuries which can be life-threatening.

(1) Elicit the history to discover evidence of a blow to the abdomen, loins or lower back.
(2) Examine carefully the abdomen, loins and lower back. Measure the girth.
(3) Rupture of an abdominal viscus may cause pain, abdominal bruising, tenderness and guarding and increasing girth, falling blood pressure, rising pulse, respiratory embarrassment.
(4) Urinary retention may cause pain or, in the semi-conscious patient, restlessness. However, do not catheterise a patient who is passing only blood *per urethram* since he may have a ruptured urethra. Instead, consult the urologist.

Gunshot wounds

Low velocity hand-gun bullets inflict wounds that can be managed by conventional surgical methods; such bullets damage only the tissue they touch. High velocity wounds from rifle bullets or explosive blast fragments have a mortality four to five times higher and require specialised attention.

The external appearance of such wounds is highly deceptive: very small entrance wounds hide extremely severe wounds with extensive necrotic tissue contaminated with clostridia spores, other bacteria, clothing and debris. To avoid gas gangrene, these wounds must be treated by excision of the damaged tissue, followed 4–5 days later by delayed primary closure and, if necessary, skin grafts. Tissue up to 30 times the volume of the projectile may need to be excised.

History

- The history may be directly relevant in revealing the cause of the injury (eg epilepsy). In children, remember the possibility of child abuse (Section 9.4).
- Drug therapy (eg corticosteroids) may influence patient management.
- Many patients involved in road traffic accidents and personal violence have been drinking alcohol (take a blood alcohol level).
- Diabetics may lapse into coma if not given their medication. Unconsciousness after a head injury is usually, but not always, caused by brain damage – consider other causes.

It is essential that every patient involved in assault or accident be examined carefully clinically and radiologically and precise records kept in the case notes. Legal sequelae are commonplace.

Infection (see Tables 8.1 and 8.2)

Meningitis

Meningitis may occur if there are dural tears, skull fractures compound to the exterior or into paranasal sinuses, or scalp wounds. Sulphonamides or rifampicin are indicated (Table 8.1). Remember to keep any patient on sulphonamides adequately hydrated (consider giving mist. pot. cit.) to avoid crystalluria.

Local infection

Infection is uncommon unless teeth are involved in the fracture line, when they may have to be removed. The main precautions are:

(1) Prompt wound toilet.
(2) Removal of foreign bodies, including fragments of teeth, from the wound.
(3) Antimicrobial prophylaxis (usually benzyl penicillin 600 mg 6-hourly IM).

Osteomyelitis (often staphylococcal) can be a complication of fractures open to the skin, particularly as a result of gunshot wounds.

Tetanus
Toxoid or antitetanic globulin should be given if the wound is contaminated and there is doubt about the patient's immunity to tetanus (Table 8.2).

8.3 Patients with maxillofacial and head injuries who should be admitted to hospital

Patients with maxillofacial injuries should be admitted to hospital if there is:

- A danger to the airway (eg laryngeal trauma, etc).
- Fracture of the skull.
- Any loss of consciousness.
- Post-traumatic amnesia.
- Serious injuries or bleeding.
- Middle third facial fracture.
- Mandibular fracture unless simple and treatable in the dental chair.
- Zygomatic fracture with, or where there is danger of, ocular damage.
- Any other reason (see Section 7.1).
- Some children with head injuries and patients living alone, without a responsible companion, and those of reduced responsibility, should also be admitted.

If patients are not admitted, *they must be warned to return to hospital if there is any deterioration in conscious level, headache, neck stiffness or vomiting*, all features suggesting neurological complications.

8.4 Priorities in operative management of patients with maxillofacial fractures

(1) Neurosurgical intervention for intracranial bleeding.
Get an urgent neurological opinion if there are any of the following:
  (*a*) Deteriorating conscious level.
  (*b*) Increasing restlessness.
  (*c*) Headache.
  (*d*) Vomiting.
  (*e*) Focal signs or fits.
  (*f*) Dilatation of pupils.
  (*g*) Bradycardia.
  (*h*) Rising blood pressure.
(2) Abdominal surgery to establish haemostasis, etc.

(3) Orthopaedic surgery.
(4) Maxillofacial surgery. Soft tissue repair; temporary fixation if needed, and then definitive care of the fractures.

8.5 Definitive management of maxillofacial fractures

Facial fractures are diagnosed primarily from the history and clinical examination (see below), supplemented where required by radiographic examination. It may be necessary to request radiographs before having the opportunity to examine the patient (Tables 1.18 and 8.4).

Facial fractures can be classified as:
● closed (simple): no skin or mucosal penetration.
● open (compound): skin or mucosal penetration (or compound into the periodontium).
● comminuted: bone fragmented, can also be simple or compound.
● greenstick: occur in children.

These may all be displaced or undisplaced, depending on the severity of the fracture, angulation of fracture, effect of muscle action, presence of erupted teeth and the intactness of the periosteum.

Table 8.4   Radiographs for maxillofacial fractures

Fracture site	Radiographs recommended initially[a]
Mandibular	Panoramic or bilateral oblique laterals Postero-anterior view of mandible (or reverse Townes) Occlusal
TMJ and condyle	Conventional and high OPT or reverse OPT Reverse Townes
Zygomatic arch	Submentovertex (exposed for zygomatic arches, not base of skull)
Middle third[b]	Occipitomental 30° Occipitomental 10° Lateral skull
Skull	Postero-anterior view of skull Lateral skull (brow up) Submentovertex (exposed for base of skull) CAT scan
Nasal	Soft tissues lateral view for nasal bones Occipitomental 30°

[a] See Table 1.18 for further details
[b] Water's view or tomograms for orbital floor fractures

Radiographs for maxillofacial and head injuries
- Occipitomental views (10° and 30°).
- Lateral skull view.
- Postero-anterior view of skull.
- Postero-anterior view of mandible.
- Oblique laterals of mandible, or panoramic view.
- CAT scans.

Specific views may also be indicated in fractures of particular bones (Table 8.4).

Information to give consultant or his deputy regarding a patient with maxillofacial injuries
- Patient's age and occupation.
- Patient's sex.
- Relevant medical history.
- Type of accident or assault.
- Whether the patient is, or has been, unconscious.
- Describe facial fractures.
- Note any other facial injuries.
- Describe state of dentition; general care and injuries.
- Describe any other injuries – particularly those which are serious.
- Describe anything which may necessitate *urgent operation*.

Other information to record
- Photographs for medicolegal purposes.
- Results of investigations.
- Treatment.

Malar fractures
Diagnosis
- History of trauma to the cheek.
- Depression of the cheek (may be masked by oedema).
- Haematoma and lateral subconjunctival haemorrhage with no posterior limit.
- Step deformities on the orbital rim. Pain on palpation.
- Restricted eye movements. Possible enophthalmos or exophthalmos.
- Infra-orbital nerve anaesthesia, hypoaesthesia or paraesthesia.
- Restriction of mandibular movements (zygoma interfering with coronoid movement).

Radiological examination (see Tables 1.18 and 8.4.)
- Fracture lines.
- Step deformities of orbital rim.
- Distracted zygomatico-frontal or zygomatico-maxillary sutures.
- Fluid in antrum.

Management
Undisplaced fractures with no ocular complications may need no treatment.

Reduction
- By elevating it from the temporal region (Gillies approach);
- By using a hook applied from the face;
- From an intra-oral approach;
- By exposing the fracture and reducing it directly.

Retention (may not be needed)
- Direct wiring.
- Pin fixation.
- Plating.
- Packing of the maxillary antrum.
- Kirschner wire.

Complications
- Malunion – leaving a cheek depressed or jaw movements restricted.
- Sensory changes over ipsilateral cheek.
- Compensation neurosis.
- Ocular complications.
    - (*a*) Periorbital oedema. Do not allow this to prevent careful examination of the eye.
    - (*b*) Periorbital surgical emphysema. Occurs when patient blows nose in fractures involving antral or nasal walls. Ensure patients avoid this.
    - (*c*) Enophthalmos. May indicate orbital blow-out.
    - (*d*) Nasolacrimal duct damage. May not appear obvious until 10 days after trauma. Fractures of medial orbital wall may damage duct and produce swelling, pain and oedema, sometimes with epiphora.
    - (*e*) Diplopia. Often caused by oedema and haemorrhage, when it settles within about 10 days. If not, this may be caused by muscle entrapment or nerve damage.
    - (*f*) Optic nerve damage. A potential cause of blindness. May be caused

by direct trauma if there is fracture of the optic foramen. Examine the consensual reflex.

(g) Retrobulbar haemorrhage. A potential cause of blindness; presents with pain, proptosis and paralysis of eye movements. Always check visual acuity. Also check as soon as the patient has regained consciousness after operation for reduction, then half-hourly for 6 hours and hourly for 12 hours.

Mandibular fractures

Diagnosis

- History of trauma to mandible.
- Pain.
- Swelling.
- Bruising (haematoma) (particularly sublingually).
- Bleeding (usually intra-orally).
- Mobility of fragments (and possible crepitus).
- Deranged occlusion.
- Paraesthesia/anaesthesia of nerves involved in the site (usually lower labial anaesthesia).

Radiological examination (see Tables 1.18 and 8.4)

- Fracture lines.
- Step deformities.
- Widening of periodontal space (if teeth are involved).

Management

- Simple undisplaced fractures may be treated conservatively with a soft diet.
- Antibiotic if tooth involved.
- Definitive treatment of displaced fractures:

(1) Reduction and fixation
(2) Prevention of infection
(3) Fixation for 4 weeks, then test for union

Retention

Indirect fixation (stabilising mandible against maxilla, intermaxillary fixation – IMF)

- Eyelet and tie wires (where there is a substantial dentition).
- Arch bar and tie wires (where several teeth are missing or there are bilateral fractures).
- Splints (cap splints on teeth, or Gunning's splint if edentulous).

Direct fixation

- Direct (transosseous) wire, on the upper or lower borders of the mandible (or mid-alveolar).
- Bone plates, eg Champey plates (now popular, since IMF not needed).
- External pin fixation.
- Internal pin fixation (eg using Kirschner wire).

Complications

Body. Deformity; limitation of movement; inadequate mastication (?malocclusion).

Condyle. Impaired growth (children); chronic traumatic arthrosis; ankylosis; limitation and abnormality of movement; dislocation; malocclusion; asymmetry of chin. Mandibular division of trigeminal nerve: anaesthesia, paraesthesia; hyperalgesia; neuralgia.

General. Infection; malunion – anatomically incorrect healing; delayed union; non-union due to a variety of local or systemic problems. Compensation neurosis.

Fractures of the middle third of the facial skeleton
Despite its inadequacies the Le Fort classification of facial fractures has persisted (fig. 8.6).

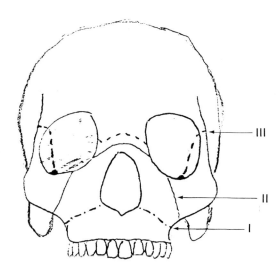

Fig. 8.6   Le Fort lines of middle third facial fractures.

Le Fort III: high level
Le Fort II: pyramidal
Le Fort I: low level or Guérin's fracture
The variations are many in different patients and on opposite sides of the mouth. They are often closed fractures.

Diagnosis
- History of severe trauma to the face, usually in a backward and downward direction (often a road traffic accident).
- Swelling of the upper lip in Le Fort I, and massive swelling of face (ballooning) in severe Le Fort II and III fractures (Panda facies).
- Pain.
- Bleeding (usually from the nose); haematoma – bilateral black eyes common; buccal sulcus also affected.
- Mobility, sometimes gross (floating face).
- Posterior gagging of occlusion and lengthening of the face (anterior open bite).
- Percussing teeth may elicit a 'cracked-pot' sound in dento-alveolar as well as in any of the Le Fort types of fracture.
- Subconjunctival ecchymoses.
- Anaesthesia of the infra-orbital nerves.
- Double vision/restricted eye movements.
- Cerebrospinal rhinorrhoea – leakage of CSF through the nose (or into nasopharynx).
- Bruising in the region of the greater palatine foramen.

Radiographic examination (see Tables 1.18 and 8.4)
These fractures are mainly diagnosed clinically. Damage to the orbital walls, floor and roof, and displacement or entrapment of orbital soft tissues is often identified using CAT scanning. Fractures around the orbital apex or medial wall may be undetectable by other means.

Management
In the minimally mobile fractured maxilla there is occasionally a place for simple IMF. Established methods of fixation and immobilisation include:

- Craniomandibular fixation (eg by means of a box-frame or halo frame).
- Craniomaxillary fixation (eg by means of supra-orbital pins and a Levant frame or internal suspension from a halo frame).
- Intermaxillary fixation using arch-bars with internal suspension from frontozygomatic wires or circumzygomatic wires to lower arch-bar.

Fixation is maintained for 3 weeks, when union is tested.

Complications

Nose. Deformity, deviation, obstruction, anosmia.

Orbit. Diplopia (muscle or fibrous entrapment/nerve injury), lacrimal duct damage, enophthalmos, optic nerve injury and/or ruptured globe, retinal damage.

Maxilla and zygomatic bones. Deformity, malocclusion, zygomatic interference with mouth opening.

Maxillary division of trigeminal nerve. Anaesthesia, paraesthesia, hyperalgesia, neuralgia.

Cerebral. CSF leak (± meningitis), headaches, aerocoele, cavernous sinus thrombosis, compensation neurosis, epilepsy.

Delayed union is occasionally encountered, with the maxilla retaining a degree of mobility (springiness) which is not in itself clinically significant. Non-union is virtually never seen.

Maxillofacial fractures: post-operative care

Care of airway

In case there is sudden and unexpected respiratory obstruction by vomiting, bleeding or oedema, have adequate suction available and, if there is IMF, wire cutters, wire holding forceps and box spanner always at the bedside in order to undo fixation, and adequate suction. Show the nurses how to remove IMF.

General observations

- Airway and respiration.
- Conscious level and neurological observations.
- Blood pressure.
- Pulse.
- Temperature.
- Fluid balance.

If there are deterioration of consciousness, behavioural changes or ophthalmic or neurological signs, obtain a neurological opinion (? aerocele; ? intracranial haemorrhage).

Specific observations

During or after elevation of a fractured zygoma or surgery around the orbit, there is a small risk of retrobulbar haemorrhage. This is an emergency; call for an ophthalmologist. Always do half-hourly observations for 6 hours then hourly for the next 12 hours. Retrobulbar haemorrhage presents with pain, proptosis, poor vision and loss of pupil reflexes.

Antimicrobials
Give penicillin for 5 days after fixation, and sulphonamide (or rifampicin) for 7 days, or until at least 2 days after the CSF leak stops (Table 8.1). If the CSF leak is still present 7–10 days after fixation of fracture, obtain a neurosurgical opinion.

Chloramphenicol eye drops 0·5% may be used if there is conjunctival damage.

Feeding
Food should be liquidised, but a dietician should be consulted to avoid a monotonous diet. The patient with IMF can feed with a straw, plastic suction tubes, etc. Clean the mouth after meals.

Oral hygiene
Blood clots and dried blood should be cleaned away with a bicarbonate mouthwash. The mouth and fixation should be cleaned gently with a soft brush. Chlorhexidine mouthwashes are valuable: 0·2% aqueous chlorhexidine at least twice daily.

Sutures, pins and screws
Do not permit crusts to remain on these. Clean with chlorhexidine and then apply Polyfax. Remove skin sutures early; clean the skin with ether, support suture lines with Steristrip or Micropore.

Fixation and splints
Check fixation and splints daily. Cover wire ends with soft wax. In middle third fractures, shorten up the maxilla at 48 hours post-operatively.

Splint removal
Indicated when union is assured. Remove splints with splint removal forceps or old extraction forceps. Remove as much cement as possible, and then clean the teeth with an ultrasonic scaler, or ask a hygienist to help.

The wider care of trauma patients
Trauma, particularly from assaults, may produce social and psychological effects which may necessitate social or psychiatric care or help from victims support schemes, especially for advice about compensation, alcohol and drug dependence, and compensation neuroses.

9

Child Dental Health and Orthodontics

9.1 Tooth eruption and development (see Table 9.1)

There is a wide variation in the timing of tooth eruption. Occasionally, eruption is delayed, most often because of a local obstruction, but is otherwise usually uncomplicated, unless by pericoronitis (Table 5.3), which is virtually restricted to lower third molars.

Teething

Many infant illnesses are blamed on teething. Tooth eruption can cause mild gingivitis and soreness and, as a consequence, irritability, disturbed sleep, dribbling, reduction of amount eaten, increased fluid intake, flushing of the cheeks, and a circum-oral rash. It cannot be blamed for high fever or convulsions.

The latter are the result of coincidental systemic disease (usually infection). An acutely sore mouth coinciding with teeth eruption is usually viral stomatitis (Table 5.3), frequently herpetic.

9.2 Fluorides

Where the water supply is not adequately fluoridated, fluorides can be administered in a mouthrinse or toothpaste, or by professional application or, best of all, as tablets or drops.

(*a*) *Mouthrinse:*

0·2% neutral sodium fluoride solution
10 ml to be rinsed for at least 1 minute, once a week
Unsuitable for children of less than 6 years old.

(*b*) *Toothpastes*

Sodium monofluorophosphate is the most widely used salt

(*c*) *Applications*

Fresh 8–10% stannous fluoride reduces caries by up to 40–50%, but stains

Table 9.1 Tooth development

	Tooth	Tooth germ fully formed	Calcification begins	Calcification of crown complete	Appearance in oral cavity	Root complete
Deciduous	Incisors	17th week foetal life	4 months foetal life	2–3 months	6–9 months	1–1·5 years after appearance in oral cavity
	Canines	18th week foetal life	5 months foetal life	9 months	16–18 months	
	1st molars	19th week foetal life	6 months foetal life	6 months	12–14 months	
	2nd molars	19th week foetal life	6 months foetal life	12 months	20–30 months	
Permanent	Incisors	30th week foetal life	3–4 months (upper lateral incisor 10–12 months)	4–5 years	Lower 6–8 years Upper 7–9 years	2–3 years after appearance in oral cavity
	Canines	30th week foetal life	4–5 months	6–7 years	Lower 9–10 years Upper 11–12 years	
	Premolars	30th week foetal life	1·5–2·5 years	5–7 years	10–12 years	
	1st molars	24th week foetal life	Birth	2·5–3 years	6–7 years	
	2nd molars	6th month	2·5–3 years	7–8 years	11–13 years	
	3rd molars	6th year	7–10 years	12–16 years	17–21 years	

teeth at restoration margins. Acidulated phosphate fluoride 1·23% applied for 4 minutes to dried teeth twice a year is preferred in many centres.

(*d*) *Tablets* (Table 9.2)

9.3 Orthodontics

Examination of the patient requiring treatment
History
- Reason for attendance and estimate of cooperation.
- Previous dental history.
- ? Family history of malocclusion ? Siblings having orthodontic treatment.
- Medical history.

Skeletal form and relationships
Skeletal class
Clinical estimate of Frankfort/mandibular plane angle
Facial asymmetry
Mandibular path of closure.

Soft tissues
Lips: form, activity, ?habitually apart or together; lip line (?control of 21|12).
Swallow: tongue thrust.
(Sucking habits and speech).

Table 9.2 Recommended fluoride supplements[a] for children at different ages, in relation to concentration of fluoride in drinking water

	Concentration of fluoride in drinking water (ppm)		
Age	< 0·3	0·3–0·7	> 0·7
2 weeks to 2 years	0·25	0	0
2–4 years	0·50	0·25	0
4–16 years	1·00	0·50	0

[a]Number of tablets, each containing 2·2 mg sodium fluoride to be taken daily (2·2 mg sodium fluoride contains 1 mg fluoride). Drops are more satisfactory for infants.

Intra-oral examination
General
  Oral hygiene, gingival condition, caries rate.
  Teeth erupted.
Incisor segments.
  Centre lines in relation to face.
  Incisor angulation ($\uparrow$to Frankfort; $\downarrow$to mandibular planes).
  Overjet (measure).
  Overbite.
  Malposition of individual teeth.
  Classify incisor relationship.
Canines
  Angulation.
  Malposition.
  If unerupted – locate (see also Table 2.3).
Buccal segments
  Malposition of individual teeth.
  Crossbites.
  Classify molar occlusion.

Radiographic examination
Account for all teeth; condition of crowns, roofs and bone

Treatment planning
Best carried out by the clinician who will do the treatment.

Extraction of teeth in children
Dental extractions usually have a profound effect upon the developing dentition. If necessary, an orthodontic opinion should be sought for non-urgent cases.

Extraction of deciduous teeth
There is seldom a case for the removal of one deciduous tooth only, unless it is close to being shed naturally, or has been retained so long that it is causing its successor to be displaced.

Enforced extractions of deciduous canines or molars should be balanced to prevent shift of centre lines. The balancing extraction need not be the contralateral tooth. A second deciduous molar extraction can be balanced by loss of the contralateral C, D or E.

The availability of orthodontic radiographs will ensure that there are no other problems (such as a mid-line supernumerary) which may also require attention (Section 1.3).

Extraction of permanent teeth
Although many orthodontic treatments include the extraction of first premolars, there may be indications for the removal of a different tooth. Particularly check the following.
At assessment:
- All successional teeth are present.
- Other teeth are of good prognosis (eg first molars).
At extraction:
- The correct tooth is written down clearly in the notes.
- The patient and parent understand that a permanent tooth is being removed.
- Parental consent has been obtained.
- Any appliance is being worn satisfactorily before orthodontic extractions are performed.

Adjustment of removable appliances
At each monthly visit confirm that:
- The appliance is comfortable.
- Oral hygiene is good.
- The appliance wear has been continuous (the posterior outline of the appliance baseplate will be seen in the mouth).
- Tooth movement has been satisfactory in amount and direction. Movement of canines should be at least a millimetre per month and, provided that the appliance is worn at mealtimes, excessive overbite should reduce at the same rate.

In addition, measure and record:
- The overjet, using a metal ruler. A general increase in overjet of more than a millimetre indicates loss of anchorage.
- The distance between the moving tooth and a convenient reference tooth, for example the distance between the canine tip and the first molar groove can be most easily recorded as pin pricks made on the patient's chart by dividers.
- The overbite (where a bite plane is being used to depress lower incisors).

9.4 The battered child
The 'battered child syndrome' (child abuse) refers to a condition in young

children, usually under the age of 3 years, who present with injuries received as a result of non-accidental violence, inflicted (usually) by a parent or guardian.

Recognition
- Inexplicable delay between injury and medical attention.
- Obvious discrepancy between the nature of the injuries and the explanation offered by the parent.
- The child is often the only one in the family to receive repeated assaults (frequently the youngest, and often unwanted or rejected).
- The child may often have been seen elsewhere or previously, for other injuries.
- Predominantly a lower social class, Anglo-American-Nordic phenomenon and, within Britain, in Irish and negroid immigrants.
- Sixty per cent recurrence: 10% eventual fatal injury.

Lesions
- Bruising, especially around the arms (child has been gripped and shaken), on the scalp and face, especially around the mouth; also around the joints of the upper limbs, neck, chest, and abdomen.
- Lacerations of upper labial mucosa, often with torn fraenum.
- Bite marks are common, on the face and upper limbs.
- Fractures of ribs, long bones (commonly at epiphyses) and skull.
- Other lesions include cigarette burns, ruptured viscera (lacerated liver, torn bowel), eye injuries, periostitis over facial bones or limbs.

Action in suspected battering
It is not enough merely to treat the acute injuries and then return the child to a dangerous domestic situation. Team-work is essential; general practitioners, health visitors, child care services, paediatricians and other medical specialists must work together.

As a temporary measure, where the parents are unwilling voluntarily to leave the child in care, a breathing space can be gained under Section 28(1) of the Children and Young Persons Act 1969. The authority of a magistrate is obtained to 'detain the child in a place of safety if there is reasonable cause to believe that his/her proper development is being avoidably prevented or neglected, or his/her health is being avoidably impaired or neglected, or he/she is being ill treated'. This authority is for a maximum time of 28 days, but allows the local Child Abuse Committee, where such an organisation has been instituted, to further investigate and discuss the child and decide upon the best course of action.

Admit the child suspected to have been non-accidentally injured under a specialist appropriate to its injuries, or under a paediatrician, for standard medical and surgical care. If the injuries do not warrant admission and the parent is not prepared to allow the child to be admitted, it is essential that the Social Services Department be contacted by the medical social worker in the hospital.

Record the history, and clinical and radiographic findings (complete skeletal survey needed). Photographs can be useful.

The child should not be discharged from hospital until appropriate enquiries have been made through the Social Services Department.

9.5 Traumatised teeth (Table 9.3)

The immediate management is shown in Table 9.3. Avulsed teeth should be handled by the crown, washed in saline or milk, and replanted as soon as possible.

9.6 Patients with cleft lip or palate

The child should be examined at birth with regard to orofacial and other possible anomalies. Interdisciplinary management with plastic surgeons, ENT surgeons, oral surgeons, orthodontists, restorative dentists and speech therapists is indicated.

Table 9.3 Management of traumatised permanent incisors

Fractures	Management
Enamel only	—
Enamel and dentine but no pulpal exposure	Calcium hydroxide (eg Dycal or Life) to protect dentine; restore crown (acid-etch composite, or crown)
Enamel and dentine with pulpal exposure but pulp vital	Partial pulpotomy
Enamel and dentine with pulpal exposure but pulp non-vital	Root canal treatment, filling, eg with Diaket
Slightly mobile teeth	Soft diet
Mobile teeth	Splint for 3–4 weeks[a]
Avulsed teeth	Replant and splint[a]. Endodontics if tooth firms up

[a] Splint with a polythene occlusal splint or metal foil or epimine resin (Scutan) or acrylic resin (eg Trim). Alternatively, acid etch and splint with composite resin ± wire strengthener; however, this is difficult to remove.

Table 9.4 Schedule for management of patients with cleft lip and palate

Approximate age	Schedule[a]
Birth	Assessment with photographs, impressions and radiographs. Discussions with team and parents. Possible presurgical orthodontics
3 months	Repair cleft lip
12–18 months	Repair cleft palate. Oral hygiene instruction to parents
30 months	Speech assessment
4 years +	Consider surgical revision of lip and/or palate
5 years +	Consider surgery for correction of speech defects. Preventive dentistry
8 years +	Simple orthodontics
10 years +	Alveolar bone graft
12 years +	Definitive orthodontics
16 years +	Maxillofacial surgery may be indicated for correction of maxillary hypoplasia or nasal deformity. Restorative dentistry

[a]Preventive dental care required throughout.

The parents must be carefully counselled as to the treatment plan and prognosis.

9.7 Orthognathic surgery

A wide range of procedures are available but Le Fort osteotomies are commonly carried out in the maxilla, sagittal split osteotomies in the mandible (figs 9.1 and 9.2). Other aspects are discussed in Chapter 7.

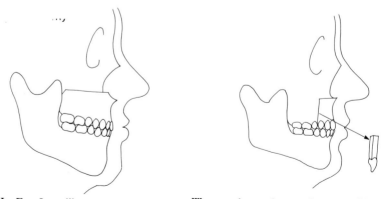

Le Fort I maxillary osteotomy   Wassmund procedure on the premaxilla

Fig. 9.1 Two examples of maxillary osteotomies. Reproduced by kind permission of Professor G. R. Seward.

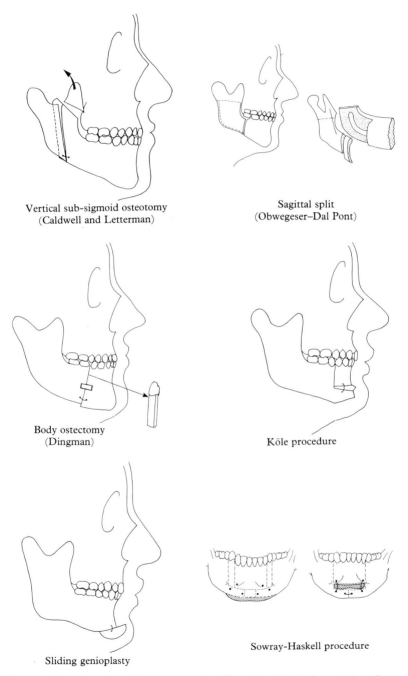

Vertical sub-sigmoid osteotomy
(Caldwell and Letterman)

Sagittal split
(Obwegeser–Dal Pont)

Body ostectomy
(Dingman)

Köle procedure

Sliding genioplasty

Sowray-Haskell procedure

Fig. 9.2 Examples of mandibular osteotomies. Reproduced by kind permission of Professor G. R. Seward.

10

Restorative dentistry

Restorative dentistry is fully discussed in several standard textbooks; the purpose of this brief chapter is to act as an aide-memoire to some aspects which can be difficult to commit fully to memory.

10.1 Management of dental hypersensitivity

Desensitise with *one* of the following:

- Sodium fluoride paste.
- Stannous fluoride gel.
- Siloxane ester coating (Tresiolan).
- Strontium chloride (Sensodyne) or formaldehyde toothpaste (Emo-form).

10.2 Management of intrinsically discoloured teeth

Many of these require no treatment, but a wide choice of procedures is available (Table 10.1).

10.3 International standard digital code

Rotary instruments are specified using a code of 15 digits; the digits sequentially represent the features shown below (fig. 10.1):

10.4 Dental cements

These are summarised in Table 10.2

10.5 Tooth coloured filling materials

Silicates
Brittle, acid soluble and acidic

Table 10.1   Management of intrinsically discoloured teeth

Management	Indications	Comments
Masterly inactivity	(1) Discoloured deciduous teeth (2) Minimal discolouration in permanent dentition	
Bleaching	Roof-filled non-vital teeth	May avoid need for crowning. Carry out under rubber dam; ensure adequate root canal seal; etch dentine with 30% phosphoric acid; degrease with 1:3 chloroform; 95% ethanol; bleach with 30% hydrogen peroxide × 2. Repeat as required.
Masking	Teeth discoloured because of an intrinsic defect	Acid-etch and composite for limited defect. Acrylic laminate veneers useful.
Crowning	Discoloured permanent teeth where above procedures inappropriate or teeth heavily restored	Excellent aesthetics. Expensive and time-consuming

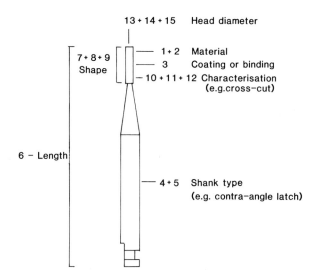

Fig. 10.1   International standard digital code for rotary instruments

Table 10.2 Dental cements

Type	Powder	Liquid	Main uses
Zinc-oxide eugenol	Zinc oxide	Eugenol	Pulp capping Cavity lining Temporary restoration
Zinc phosphate	Zinc oxide	Phosphoric acid	Cavity lining cement
Zinc polycarboxylate or polyacrylate	Zinc oxide	Polyacrylic acid	Cement

Silicate	Aluminosilicate
	   (contains fluoride)
		Phosphoric acid	Tooth-coloured
			   restoration

Glass ionomer	Aluminosilicate
	   (contains fluoride)
		Polyacrylic or
		   polymaleic acid
			Restoration of
			   deciduous teeth
			Cervical restorations
			   cement

Glass ionomers

Adhere to prepared dentine: less soluble and acidic than silicates, but must be kept dry during setting

Polymethyl methacrylate

Good initial aesthetics but high shrinkage and low abrasion resistance leading to staining

Composites

- Low shrinkage, good colour stability
- Based on polymethylmethacrylate or diacrylate and activated chemically or by light source.
- Short working time for chemically-activated types. Ultra-violet light activated types have long working time but there is some light hazard. White-light activated types have shorter working time.
- Microfine types are easier to polish than others.
- Avoid using metal instruments and eugenol-containing cements.

10.6 Clinical indices of periodontal disease

Though several indices are available, commonly used indices are shown in Table 10.3.

Table 10.3   Clinical indices of periodontal disease

Index	Sites assessed	Score
Debris	6 | 1 4 4 1 | 6 Buccal and lingual	0 = no plaque 1 = < 1/3 surface covered 2 = > 1/3 < 2/3 surface covered 3 = > 2/3 surface covered
Bleeding	6 | 1 4 4 1 | 6 Buccal and lingual	0 = No bleeding on blunt probing 1 = Bleeding only 30 seconds after blunt probing 2 = Immediate bleeding on probing 3 = spontaneous bleeding

10.7 Periodontal surgery techniques

Surgery is contra-indicated unless oral hygiene is adequate. Techniques are summarised in Table 10.4

10.8 Surgical treatment of gingival and periodontal disease

Pocket elimination

Scaling and root-planning unless the pocket is inaccessible to this or deeper than 6 mm. Inverse bevel flap is generally the most appropriate.

Mucogingival problems

In selected situations:

- Fraenal interference: fraenectomy
- Recession or cleft: gingival graft

Table 10.4   Periodontal surgical techniques

Procedure	Type
Subgingival curettage	Reattachment
Gingivectomy	Resection
Reverse bevel gingivectomy	Resection
Excisional new attachment procedure	Reattachment
Inverse bevel flap (modified Widman)	Reattachment
Apically repositioned flap	Reposition

- Where repositioning indicated, apically repositioned flap
- Gingival cleft – laterally repositioned flap

Gingival hyperplasia and false pocketting
Gingivectomy/gingivoplasty

10.9 Possible contra-indications to fixed prostheses

- Diastemas
- Unrestored abutments
- Compromised abutments
- Caries susceptibility
- Susceptibility to periodontal disease
- Inadequate occlusal clearance

10.10 Preprosthetic surgery

Osseous procedures
- Alveoloplasty
- Mylohyoid ridge reduction
- Removal of bony prominences
- Tuberoplasty
- Osseointegrated and other implants
- Ridge augmentation

Soft tissue procedures
- Fraenectomy
- Tuberosity reduction
- Vestibuloplasty —
  - (a) submucous
  - (b) supraperiosteal with skin graft.

10.1 Materials for repair of bone defects or ridge augmentation
Some of these are shown in Table 10.5.

10.12 Dental implants
Various endosseous implants are now available (the main ones are listed in Table 10.6).

Table 10.5   Materials for repair of bone defects or for ridge augmentation

	Type	Comments
Autogenous bone	Intra oral origin	Limited material available
	Extra oral origin	Two operations required
Allograft bone	Donor Cadaver Freeze-dried	Possibility of infection or rejection
Xenograft bone	Usually porcine	Limited success
Ceramics	Hydroxyapatite Tricalcium phosphate	Biocompatible but hydroxyapatite must be in crystalline ceramic (sintered) form, or it is resorbed rapidly. Useful for alveolar ridge augmentation or repair of infra bony defects
Plaster of Paris		Resorbed rapidly

Merits of osseo-integrated implants

Advantages
- Independent of adjacent teeth
- Prosthesis is retentive

Table 10.6   Main implants in current use

Type	Comments
Subperiosteal	Rests on bone surface, beneath periosteum. Bone must be exposed surgically for direct impression. Implant is fabricated for individual patient. Most suitable for completely edentulous mandible
Transosteal (staple bone plate)	Penetrates inferior border of mandible and projects through ridge mucosa. Skin incision required. Vitallium or gold implants
Endosseous	Embedded in maxillary or mandibular bone and projects through ridge mucosa. Cylindrical threaded endosteal osseo-integrated titanium implant is the version of most proven success (Bränemark: Nobelpharma) Many variations available, for example: Nobelpharma TPS (titanium plasma spray) screws ITI IMZ hollow baskets Implants may also be ceramic-based (eg Tübingen)

- Aesthetic
- Immune to caries

Disadvantages
- Invasive: surgery is required
- Time-consuming and costly
- Need an adequate amount of bone

Contra-indications for osseo-integrated implants (Table 10.7)
- Lack of adequate training of operator.
- Poor patient motivation, or psychiatric disease.
- Poor patient oral hygiene.
- Inadequate minimum requirements for quantity or quality of bone.
- Systemic conditions, eg pregnancy, local radiotherapy, immunocompromised patient; alcoholism or drug abuse, susceptibility to infective endocarditis.
- Hypersensitivity to components of implants.

Criteria for success of implants*
- Bone loss no greater than one third of the vertical height of the implant and rate loss less than 0·2 mm annually after 1st year.
- Good occlusal balance and vertical dimension.
- Gingival inflammation amenable to treatment.
- Mobility < 1 mm in any direction.
- Absence of symptoms of infection.
- Absence of damage to adjacent teeth.
- Absence of paraesthesia, anaesthesia or violation of inferior dental canal, antrum or nasal passage.
- No evidence of peri-implant radiolucency.

10.13 Denture care (see Table 10.8)
Summary of recommendations:

New complete dentures:
Use a soft brush and soap combined with a twice-weekly soak in a hypochlorite solution.

---

*After Bolender C L. *J Dent Educ* 1988; **52**: 757–759.

Table 10.7   Indications and contra-indications for different implants

| Site | Indicated implant | | Contra-indicated implant |
	Definite	Possible	
Edentulous mandible	Subperiosteal: 50–70 years of age; placed on basal bone opposing complete denture Transosteal (staple): Adults 9 mm + vertical bone height Endosseous (Bränemark): 7 mm + vertical bone height and 6 mm + bone width	Core-vent. IMZ	Blades Ramus frame
Partial edentulous anterior mandible			Subperiosteal Transosteal
Partially edentulous posterior mandible	None	Endosseous (Bränemark): 7 mm + vertical bone height and 6 mm + bone width Core-vent IMZ	
Edentulous maxilla	Endosseous (Bränemark) 7 mm + bone height and 6 mm + bone width and favourable quality	Core-vent IMZ	Subperiosteal Blades
Partially edentulous anterior maxilla			
Partially edentulous posterior maxilla	None	Endosseous (Bränemark) 7 mm + bone height and 6 mm bone width and favourable quality Core-vent IMZ	Subperiosteal

After Bolender CL. *J Dent Educ* 1988; **52:** 757–759.

Table 10.8 Cleansing of dentures and other prostheses

	Advantages	Disadvantages
Mechanical methods		
Soap	Effective cleaning of new dentures. Denture pastes are satisfactory cleansers. A paste containing poly (methyl methacrylate) + fluoride is recommended for those with partial dentures and natural teeth	Will not remove established stain or calculus
Powders		Abrasive
Immersion methods		
Hypochlorite solutions	Some will remove stain and plaque when used as an overnight denture soak and do not bleach acrylic or damage soft linings or tissue conditioners	Most corrode cobalt-chromium and produce black discoloration with surface erosion Household solutions may bleach dentures
Alkaline peroxide	May not fulfil their promise since they will remove deposits but not calculus They do not corrode cobalt-chromium or damage soft linings	May cause deterioration of tissue-conditioning materials
Acid solutions	May render calculus amenable to mechanical removal	May corrode cobalt-chromium or damage fabrics

Old dentures:

For old dentures with deposits of stain and calculus, use a proprietary cleaner as necessary, then regular hypochlorite soaks.

Partial dentures:

Clean with a brush.

11

General Information about Employment

11.1 Applying for a new appointment

Advertisements for dental posts appear mainly in the professional journals, such as the *British Dental Journal*, *Lancet* and *British Medical Journal* or, in other countries the state or national dental journals. Discussions with colleagues and your chief will indicate when jobs are likely to appear. The more junior a hospital post, the more predictable the time of its advertisement. If you are really interested in a specific post, check the journals of the previous year to assess the time it is likely to be advertised. There may be only a very brief time between the advertisement and the closing date for applications. (If the closing date has passed, no harm is done by telephoning, as they may have had no applicants. Alternatively, your chief may suggest that this is better done by him.) Before applying for a post, ask the advice of your chief; do not just announce your firm intent to apply.

Application procedures are usually given in the advertisement. Apart from the necessary application forms, submit a curriculum vitae (see below) with a handwritten, neat and courteous letter of application.

It is also good manners to contact your referees, preferably by letter, when you have decided to apply, even though many referees will happily give a reference without a prior request. Referees may well be able to advise upon the advantages or otherwise of the advertised position and the appropriateness or otherwise of the application. They may know of another, more appropriate job. Send your referees a *recent* curriculum vitae; this will help to remind them of all your qualifications, and allow them to do you justice!

Curriculum vitae (*CV*)

The curriculum vitae is an essential component of most applications. The object is to summarise the qualifications and experience relevant to the post advertised. Brevity, clarity and honesty are required; although the format is flexible, an example is given below. Keep the CV updated.

Contents of the CV:
- Personal details (name, date of birth, sex, marital status, nationality, address)
- Secondary education (only for junior posts)
- University education
- Postgraduate education
- Diplomas of Higher Training
- University qualifications
- Distinctions
- Academic awards and honours
- Research awards
- Teaching experience
- Professional experience
  - (*a*) Hospital appointments
  - (*b*) General practice
  - (*c*) Other
- Membership of societies
- Committee assignments
- Research interests and research grants
- Contributions to specific meetings
- Published work
  - (*a*) Original reports
  - (*b*) Review papers
  - (*c*) Theses
  - (*d*) Books
  - (*e*) Chapters in books
  - (*f*) Monographs
  - (*g*) Non-printed materials
  - (*h*) Published abstracts
  - (*i*) Papers in press
  - (*j*) Papers submitted for publication
- Hobbies and outside interests

11.2 Before the interview

'Forewarned is forearmed'. Find out about the staff qualifications and publications (from colleagues, and from the *Index to Dental Literature* or *Index Medicus*).

Arrange a visit. This will give you a chance (*a*) to find out about the clinical and other responsibilities and potential of the post, (*b*) to meet potential colleagues and find out about their professional interests (try and meet all the persons with whom you hope to work), and (c) to determine conditions of service such as duty rotas, study leave, holidays, accommodation (do not leave this until you are interviewed!). It will also give the staff a chance to assess you as a potential colleague. Avoid telling them how suitable you think you are! Do not canvass (solicit for preferential treatment). Try and meet the person you are replacing, as he or she is likely to have the most useful information about the job.

Never be dissuaded from applying by rumours about possible better applicants. Competitors may fail to arrive for interview, may suffer from a drawback of which you are unaware, may interview badly, or even withdraw after appointment. Many a candidate who was destined (on the grapevine) for assured success has failed at interview!

If you are short-listed, you may need to revisit to clear up any points you are unclear about, but be careful not to appear to canvass.

11.3 At the interview

Few applicants enjoy being interviewed (even your apparently relaxed competitors), but a well-prepared applicant invariably finds the ordeal less harrowing and is often more successful. The articles by C. M. Hogg in *Dental Practice* (May–June, 1989) are well worth reading.

Arrive early: a previous candidate may have withdrawn or the interviews may be progressing more rapidly than expected. If there is a problem in attending, make every effort to communicate with the principal, head of department and/or administrator to explain.

Although there are no regulations concerning dress or personal appearance for an interview, most of the interviewers will be middle-aged or older and are often fairly conservative in their views. Ignore this if you do not care for the job (fig. 11.1).

Think beforehand about obvious questions such as:
'Why do you want this particular job?'
'Where do you see your future career?'
'Why did you take the job at your last hospital or practice?'
'When do you intend to take the ——— examination?'
'How do you see your role in relation to ——— (specific) members of staff?'
'What publications are you preparing?'
'What do you do in your spare time?'

The interview is not designed to upset or embarrass the applicant (although it may on occasion do so), but is aimed at finding the most suitable person for the post. The main purpose is not simply to gain factual information about the applicant (this is on the application form or

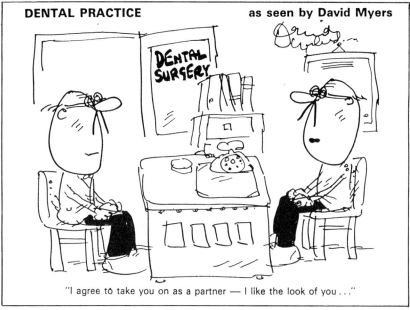

"I agree tó take you on as a partner — I like the look of you . . ."

Courtesy of D. Myers and *Dental Practice*.

Fig. 11.1

curriculum vitae), but is often the only opportunity to assess the applicant's ideas, personality and ability to relate to colleagues. These are important factors, particularly in a clinical post, and are often more important than academic factors. Act naturally, but be honest and courteous. Discuss points but never argue; you may win the battle, but you will surely lose the war.

The interview committee consists of a range of individuals, each with their own personal and professional backgrounds, experiences, interests and prejudices. A hospital or university interview committee usually consists of the head of department, other dental and/or medical specialists, representatives of the Health Authority, administration and often university. There may also be lay members and representatives of the Higher Training bodies present.

Any interview committee will have knowledge of the applicant by virtue of the:

● application letter and form;

- curriculum vitae;
- references.

Certain members will have additional information from:

- personal discussions with colleagues who have worked with the applicant;
- personal observation of the applicant, at meetings, when visiting, etc.
- the grapevine

Therefore, be sure your sins will catch up with you!

Many interviews will culminate with the question: 'Have you anything you would wish to ask us about the advertised post?' Think beforehand about a brief reply to this, remembering that, for example, you might not have located the local medical library or Postgraduate Centre on your visit (of course you knew it existed), or discussed the opportunity to attend specific dental or medical clinics that may help your education. Do not, at this time, ask about pay, study leave, time off, or holidays. You should have discussed this before the interview.

In general, be prepared to accept the post straight away if an offer is made immediately after the interview. For some posts, someone will write subsequently to the candidates to give the result of the appointment procedure. If this mechanism is adopted, it is particularly bad form to decline an offered post at this stage. At all times, if applying for more than one post, be frank and have a clear idea of which is your preferred post. Remember the grapevines!

11.4 If accepted for a position

- Thank your referees; you will need their references again.
- Ensure that your subscriptions to professional bodies and medical insurance are paid.
- Contact the clinic before taking up the post, to determine when they expect you to arrive, where to report to, and whether there are any duties to perform before or shortly after the post is taken up. Ask whether there is a specific booklet about the clinic, department and/or hospital.
- Find out your timetable and any on-call duties. If 'on-call', establish which wards, patients, and other duties are your responsibility.
- Discuss with the ward sister or senior practice nurse the best times to visit. This will often expedite the carrying out of the duties.
- A member of staff who appears promptly on the first day of a post and is well versed in protocol and responsibilities is obviously better received than one who arrives late and disorientated.

- Always wear either a clean clinical coat or gown, and look smart.
- Familiarise yourself with the layout and introduce yourself to those with whom you will be working and those who will need to recognise your signature, eg technicians or, in hospital, departments such as radiology, pharmacy and pathology.
- Find out about emergency procedures and where the emergency kits are kept on day one.

11.5 Being a successful member of staff

There is much more to being a successful member of staff than simply knowing all about dentistry, although, clearly, staff should be well-informed.

There is much truth in the saying that the three As are important in making a successful dental surgeon (and note the order!): *availability*, *affability* and *ability*.

Communication

Communication is essential in any teamwork; if it fails, this can lead to endless problems. If in doubt, ask for advice. Unless you have instructions to the contrary, contact the next most senior colleague.

The golden rules are:

- Always answer your bleep/page/phone.
- If in doubt – ask.
- Always err on the side of overcommunication.
- It is *your* duty to inform your colleagues of your whereabouts, holidays, etc.

Reliability

There is nothing more irritating than an unreliable member of staff. Reliability includes not only good timekeeping, but also reliability in case note-keeping, carrying out duties, etc. It is of paramount importance always to make legible, accurate, dated and signed records in the case notes whenever you check a patient, or when there is an incident involving a patient (eg complaint or accident) (see Section 1.7).

Keep a note book with a separate page for each patient, and the details of various procedures. In addition, ensure that you:

(a) enter details of any examination, medication or procedure, patient complaint or discharge;
(b) file all results of investigations *in the correct place*;

(c) *Do not* lose records, hide records, or take them away from where they should be.

Referrals
All patients in the hospital service must be in the charge of a consultant, who has personal responsibility for the patient, despite any delegation of duties to other professional staff. Junior staff must ensure that the consultant knows about patients admitted or seen under him, and you should not refer patients to another firm unless there is an emergency or you have been instructed to do so by your consultant or his deputy.

Off-duty rotas
Proper cover must be arranged for patients, even when the member of staff is out of the clinic and off duty. This is a clear *moral* responsibility, if not a legal one. When handing over to a colleague, be sure to indicate all patients who may require attention, preferably leaving a written list.

Hospital annual and study leave
After you have discussed this with your consultant(s), send an Annual/Study Leave form (obtainable from the hospital administrator) to the medical personnel department, as far in advance as possible of the proposed period of leave. Make it clear, in writing, exactly who has agreed to cover your duties when needed.

Interpersonal relationships
Apart from the obvious need for a good 'bedside manner' with patients, the dental surgeon must behave in a way that is acceptable to other staff and engenders their support. Communication, courtesy and consideration are essential qualities.

Behaviour towards patients
The psychological welfare of the patient must always be considered, and this is best accomplished by the personal interest and presence of the dentist, largely learnt by example and experience. Remember that words and manners may well have great significance to patients. Casual remarks will be analysed and repeated verbatim and phrases may be recalled for a lifetime. The smallest word of encouragement may well lift a patient from despair, or, conversely, lack of compassion may compound their misery. Routine is a fertile soil for indifference, but there is nothing routine for patients about their visits to, or time in, a clinic or hospital, and in their view there is no such thing as a 'minor' procedure.

The reputation of and confidence in the practice, department or hospital, as far as patients are concerned, depend largely upon the attitudes and behaviour of the staff.

Private patients

Private patients are usually affable, appreciative and cooperative. A minority are 'difficult', a few highly demanding and unreasonable. In any event, make a concerted effort to give the quality of care that you would to any patient and do not be pushed into doing anything against your better judgement. Do not mix private treatment with health service care.

Behaviour towards colleagues and staff

The new graduate is the most junior member of a team and should be ready to ask questions, but slow to offer opinions or advice. If you consider that seniors are in error (and they might be), use the utmost tact when airing this view; do not argue in front of a patient. The time to be most cautious is when feeling most confident; if in doubt, call for an opinion from a senior colleague. You are the least experienced member, even if you are brighter than other staff.

It is particularly important to avoid criticism of another practitioner. *Always* be honest, but do not speak while another clinician is talking with a patient.

Nursing staff

Most disagreements with nurses arise because of different priorities. Almost invariably there will have been an avoidable failure in communication. The following considerations should minimise potential trouble:

- The senior nurse or Sister is responsible for running the clinic, practice or ward (everything from housekeeping and equipment maintenance to administering treatment). This is particularly so in allocating duties to nurses and domestic staff. The junior dentist interferes in these matters at his own peril. Avoid telling nurses what to do. If you need assistance, politely ask the Sister or senior nurse. The obvious exception is in the case of an emergency.
- Most senior nurses respond to politeness, and are usually willing to impart their considerable knowledge and experience if you ask for advice.
- Senior nurses often regard their clinics or wards as they would their own house. Visitors, including dental staff, should observe normal social protocol; always ask permission of the nurse in charge if you wish to see a patient, do a ward round, or show a visitor around.

- A word of appreciation costs nothing.
- Excessive familiarity with the nursing staff in your own unit is most unwise.

Telephonists and receptionists
Good communications are essential in any establishment. Answer the 'page' or 'bleep' and telephone calls promptly. Receptionists and telephonists talk to everyone and can damage your reputation more quickly than anybody else if they so choose.

Secretaries and administrative staff
Secretaries are not impressed by the member of staff who 'knows it all' or criticises others. Secretaries often speak freely with senior staff, who may value their comments about junior staff, especially at reference time!

Students
New graduates should recall their immediate past when dealing with old colleagues and, in spite of what they might like to think, there is only a marginal difference in experience and knowledge. There is no need for arrogance.

Other ancillary staff
Establish at an early stage the responsibilities of and type of work carried out by ancillary staff. *Hygienists*, for example, work only to the prescription of a registered dentist and carry out oral hygiene instruction, scaling, and application of fissure sealants. *Dental therapists* can carry out simple fillings and exodontia. They are permitted to give local anaesthetic injections by infiltration, but are not permitted to give regional anaesthesia, ie inferior dental blocks.

11.6 Leaving a post

- Complete and return outstanding case notes.
- Hand in books and keys.
- Thank your consultant or principal and request him as a future referee.
- Leave a forwarding address.

11.7 Administrative points

Terms and conditions of service. A copy of the Terms and Conditions of Service of Medical and Dental Staff should be available in the Medical Personnel Department.

Contracts of employment. Employers are required to give employees, not later than 13 weeks after employment has begun, written information about their main terms of employment (Contracts of Employment Act, 1963).

Staff health. Friendly, unofficial arrangements may lead to ethical problems. Treat staff only on a formal basis, and keep proper records.

Removal expenses for hospital posts. Details of eligibility and entitlement to assistance with house purchase and removal expenses are available from the Medical Personnel Department.

Personal property and valuables. Although health authorities are not responsible for the loss or theft of personal effects, they are often insured against some risks, up to certain limits. Honorary staff not remunerated by the hospital are excluded from these arrangements.

Reimbursement of telephone rental. Staff required to participate in formal 'on-call' rotas from home on a regular basis may be eligible to reclaim costs of telephone rental. The amount that can be claimed will cover the cost of installation or reconnection and the quarterly rental on the *basic* instrument, plus VAT. Requests for inclusion on the district list of official telephone users should be written to the district administrator, supported by the head of department or consultants. Telephone accounts must have been previously settled and the receipt then submitted to the health authority.

Jury service. Under Section 32 of the Dentists Act, 1957, a dentist may be exempt from serving on all juries and inquests. Exemption must formally be obtained, and not assumed.

Witnessing of wills. Members of the administration should normally act as witnesses when a hospital patient wishes to make a will, although members of the dental staff may do so in an emergency.

Press enquiries. Routine enquiries about a hospital patient's condition are answered by the Hospital Administrator during office hours and the duty nursing officer out of hours. Do not answer enquiries yourself.

Appendices

Some commonly used symbols, abbreviations and acronyms in UK dentistry

Normal male	□	Affected male	■
Normal female	○	Affected female	●

Mating

Parents with son
and daughter
(in order of birth)

Female with
children by
two males

Propositus

Dead

Abortion or stillbirth
of unspecified sex

Annotation of family trees

AAFB	Acid- and alcohol-fast bacillus (tuberculosis)	**ADH**	Antidiuretic hormone
		ADP	Association for denture prosthesis
Ab	Antibody	**AF**	Atrial fibrillation
ACTH	Adrenocorticotrophic hormone	**Ag**	Antigen
		AGN	Acute glomerulonephritis

AI	Aortic incompetence	**CAC**	Chronic atrophic candidosis
AIDS	Acquired immune deficiency syndrome	**CAH**	Chronic active hepatitis
ALK PASE	Alkaline phosphatase	**CAT scan**	Computerised axial tomography
ALL	Acute lymphatic leukaemia	**CBC**	Complete blood count
ALT	Alanine transaminase	**CCF**	Congestive cardiac failure
AML	Acute myeloid leukaemia		
ANK	Appointment not kept	**c/c**	Completed case
ANF	Antinuclear factor	**CCU**	Coronary care unit
APTT	Activated partial thromboplastin time	**CDH**	Congenital dislocation of the hip
ARC	AIDS-related complex	**CDO**	Chief Dental Officer
ARF	Acute renal failure	**CFHIPOV**	Cleared from head injury point of view
ARV	AIDS retrovirus		
AS	Aortic stenosis	**CFT**	Complement fixation test
ASD	Atrial septal defect	**CHD**	Congenital heart disease
ASOT	Antistreptolysin O titre	**CHF**	Congestive heart failure
AST	Aspartate transaminase	**CLL**	Chronic lymphoid leukaemia
ATS	Antitetanus serum		
AV	Arteriovenous	**CLP**	Cleft lip–palate
		CMC	Chronic mucocutaneous candidosis
BCG	Bacille Calmette Guerin (vaccine against TB)	**CMI**	Cell-mediated immunity
		CML	Chronic myeloid leukaemia
BDA	British Dental Association (also British Diabetic Association)	**CMV**	Cytomegalovirus
		CNS	Central nervous system
		CO	Complaining of
BMMP	Benign mucous membrane pemphigoid	**COAD**	Chronic obstructive airways disease
BNF	*British National Formulary*	**COCET**	Committee on Dental Continuing Education and Training
BP	Blood pressure		
BPC	*British Pharmacopoeia*	**CPC**	Clinicopathological conference
BPMF	British Postgraduate Medical Federation	**CPK**	Creatine phosphokinase
		CPME	Council for Postgraduate Medical Education
B₂m	Beta 2 microglobulin		
BRA	Bite raising appliance	**CPR**	Cardiopulmonary resuscitation
BS	Behçet syndrome		
BSL	Blood sugar level	**CRF**	Chronic renal failure
BSR	British standard ratio (prothrombin index)	**CREST**	see **CRST**
		CRST	Calcinosis, Raynaud's, scleroderma, telangiectasia
BW	Bitewing		
		CSF	Cerebrospinal fluid
C	Complement	**CSSD**	Central sterile supplies department
Ca	Cancer (Ca⁺⁺ = calcium)		

CT scan	Computerised axial tomography	**DSASTAB**	DSA standards and training advisory board
CV	Curriculum vitae	**DT**	Delirium tremens
CVA	Cerebrovascular accident	**DTETAB**	Dental technicians education and training advisory board
CVP	Central venous pressure		
CVS	Cardiovascular system		
CWR	Cardiolipin Wasserman reaction	**DVT**	Deep vein thrombosis
CXR	Chest x-ray	**DXR**	Deep x-ray radiation
		EACA	Epsilon aminocaproic acid
dB	Decibels		
DDAVP	Desmopressin	**EB**	Epidermolysis bullosa
DEAC	Dental Education Advisory Committee (Dental Deans)	**EBDSA**	Examining board for DSA
		EBV	Epstein-Barr virus
DEB	Dental Estimates Board	**ECG**	Electrocardiogram
DH	Delayed hypersensitivity *or* Dermatitis herpetiformis	**ECM**	External cardiac massage
		ECT	Electroconvulsive therapy
DH	Department of Health	**EDH**	Enrolled dental hygienist
DHA	District Health Authority	**EDT**	Enrolled dental therapist
DHSS	Department of Health and Social Services (now DH)	**EDTA**	Ethylene diamine tetra-acetate
		EEG	Electroencephalogram
DIC	Disseminated intravascular coagulation	**EM**	Erythema migrans *or* erythema multiforme
		EMAS	Employment Medical Advisory Service
DIF	Direct immunofluorescence		
DLA	Dental Laboratories Association	**EMG**	Electromyogram
		EMU	Early morning urine
DLE	Discoid lupus erythematosus	**ERCP**	Endoscopic retrograde cholangiopancreato-graphy
DMFT	Decayed, missing or filled teeth		
		ES	Extra systoles
DMFS	Decayed, missing or filled surfaces	**ESR**	Erythrocyte sedimentation rate
DMT	District medical team		
DNA	Did not attend	**FB**	Foreign body
DPA	Dental practice advisor	**FBC**	Full blood count
DPB	Dental practice board	**FDP**	Fibrin degradation products
DPF	*Dental Practitioners Formulary*		
		Fe	Iron
DPT	Diphtheria, pertussis, tetanus (vaccine)	**FEV**	Forced expiratory volume
DRS	Dental reference service	**FH**	Family history
DS	Disseminated sclerosis	**FPC**	Family Practitioner Committee
DSA	Dental surgery assistant		

FRC	Forced residual capacity	**HIV**	Human immunodeficiency virus(es)
FTA	Fluorescent treponemal antibody (test)		
FTI	Free thyroxine index	**HLA**	Human leukocyte antigen
		HMEC	Hospital Medical Executive Council
		HOCM	Hypertrophic obstructive cardiomyopathy
GA	General anaesthesia		
Gamma GT	γ glutamyl transpeptidase	**HPI**	History of present illness
G6PD	Glucose-6-phosphate dehydrogenase	**HPC**	History of present complaint
GDC	General Dental Council	**HPV**	Human papillomavirus
GDP	General Dental Practitioner	**HS**	House surgeon
		HSC	Health and Safety Commission
GDPA	General Dental Practitioners Association	**HSE**	Health and Safety Executive
GDSC	General Dental Services Committee	**HSV**	Herpes simplex virus
		HTLV	Human T cell lymphotrophic virus (HTLV-III = HIV)
GFR	Glomerular filtration rate		
GGT	Gamma glutamyl transpeptidase	**HU**	Herpetiform ulcers
GIT	Gastrointestinal tract	**Hz**	Herz
GM	Grand mal		
GMH	General medical history		
GP	General practitioner		
GPI	General paralysis of the insane	**IA**	Intra-arterial
		IC	Immune complex
GTT	Glucose tolerance test	**ICU**	Intensive care unit
GU	Genito-urinary	**ICP**	Intracranial pressure
GVHD	Graft-versus-host disease	**IDD**	Insulin-dependent diabetes
		IF	Immunofluorescence *or* intrinsic factor
HANE	Hereditary angioneurotic edema (oedema)	**IHD**	Ischaemic heart disease
HAV	Hepatitis A virus	**Ig**	Immunogloblin (eg IgG, IgA, IgM, IgE)
Hb	Haemoglobin		
HbS	Haemoglobin S (Sickle-cell)	**IIF**	Indirect immunofluorescence
HBD	Hydroxybutyrate dehydrogenase	**IM**	Intramuscular
		IMF	Intermaxillary fixation
HBcAg	Hepatitis B core antigen	**INR**	International normalised ratio (*see* BSR)
HBeAg	Hepatitis B 'e' antigen	**ITU**	Intensive treatment unit
HBsAg	Hepatitis B surface antigen	**IV**	Intravenous
		IVC	Inferior vena cava
HBV	Hepatitis B virus	**IVP**	Intravenous pyelography
HDL	High density lipoproteins	**IVU**	Intravenous urogram
HDV	Hepatitis D virus		

JC	Jacob Creutz field disease	LP	Lumbar puncture *or* lichen planus
JCHTD	Joint Committee for Higher Training in Dentistry	LVF	Left ventricular failure
		LVH	Left ventricular hypertrophy
JDC	Joint Dental Committee (of MRC, DH, SERC, SHMD)	MAOI	Monoamine oxidase inhibitors
JVP	Jugular venous pressure	MaRAS	Major aphthae
		MCH	Mean corpuscular haemoglobin
KCCT	Kaolin cephalin clotting time	MCHC	Mean corpuscular haemoglobin concentration
KPTT	Kaolin partial thromboplastin time	MCV	Mean corpuscular volume
KS	Kaposi's sarcoma	MDU	Medical Defence Union
		MEA	Multiple endocrine adenoma
LA	Local anaesthesia/analgesia	MG	Myasthenia gravis
LAD	Linear IgA disease	MI	Myocardial infarct *or* mitral incompetence
LAS	Lymphadenopathy syndrome	Mini-hep	Subcutaneous heparin
LATS	Long-acting thyroid stimulator	MiRAS	Minor aphthae
LAV	Lymphadenopathy-associated virus (HIV)	MLSO	Medical laboratory scientific officer
LBBB	Left bundle branch block	MMP	Mucous membrane pemphigoid
LDC	Local Dental Committee	MND	Motor neurone disease
LDH	Lactic dehydrogenase	MPP	Mandibular pain-dysfunction
LDL	Low density lipoproteins		
LE	Lupus erythematosus	MPS	Medical Protection Society
LFH	Left femoral hernia	MRC	Medical Research Council
LFT	Liver function tests (usually serum bilirubin plus several 'liver enzymes' such as AST and GGT)	MRI	Magnetic resonance imaging
LGV	Lymphogranuloma venereum	MS	Multiple sclerosis *or* mitral stenosis
LH	Luteinising hormone	MSU	Mid-stream urine
LHF	Left heart failure		
LIH	Left inguinal hernia		
LIF	Left iliac fossa	NAD	No abnormality detected
LKKS	Liver, kidneys, spleen	NANB(H)	Non A, non B hepatitis
LLSD	Lower labial set down	NCVQ	National Council for Vocational Qualifications
LMN	Lower motor neurone		
LMP	Last menstrual period		

NHL	Non-Hodgkin's lymphoma	**PDA**	Patent ductus arteriosus
NHS	National Health Service	**PE**	Pulmonary embolism
NHSTA	National Health Service Training Authority	**PEN V**	Penicillin V
NIDD	Non insulin dependent diabetes	**PERLA**	Pupils equal reacting to light and accommodation (ie normal)
NJC	National Joint Council for the Craft of Dental Technicians	**PET**	Pre-eclamptic toxaemia (in pregnancy)
NMR	Nuclear magnetic resonance (= MRI)	**PGL**	Persistent generalised lymphadenopathy
NP	Proper name (of drug)	**Pgy**	Pregnancy
NRPB	National Radiation Protection Board	**PHT**	Pulmonary hypertension
NSAIDS	Non-steroidal anti-inflammatory drugs	**PLS**	Persistent lymphadenopathy syndrome
NSU	Non-specific urethritis	**PM**	Petit mal
NTN	No treatment needed	**PMH**	Past medical history
NTR	No treatment required	**PMNR**	Periadenitis mucosa necrotica recurrens
		POC	Polythene occlusal cover
O	Orally	**Po₂**	Partial pressure of oxygen
OA	Osteo-arthritis	**POMR**	Problem orientated medical reports
OAF	Oro-antral fistula *or* osteoclast activating factor	**PR**	Per rectum *or* pulse rate
OI	Opportunistic infection	**PRIST**	Paper radioimmunosorbent test
OM	Occipitomental (radiograph)	**PS**	Pulmonary stenosis
OPT	Orthopantomograph	**PSA**	Pleomorphic salivary adenoma
ORF	Orthograde root filling	**PSE**	Porto-systemic encephalopathy (in liver failure)
P	Wave on ECG *or* pulse	**PT**	Prothrombin time
PA	Pernicious anaemia, periapical *or* postero-anterior (radiograph)	**PTH**	Parathyroid hormone
		PUO	Pyrexia of unknown origin
PAN	Polyarteritis nodosa	**PV**	Per vaginam (or pemphigus vulgaris)
PBC	Primary biliary cirrhosis		
PCA	Patient cancelled appointment	**PWA**	Person with AIDS
PCP	Pneumocystis carinii pneumonia	**Q**	Wave on ECT
PCV	Packed cell volume		
Pco₂	Partial pressure of carbon dioxide	**R**	Wave on ECT *or* respiration

RA	Rheumatoid arthritis *or* relative analgesia	**SGPT**	*see* ALT
RAS	Recurrent aphthous stomatitis	**SHHD**	Scottish Home and Health Dept.
RAST	Radioallergosorbent test	**SHO**	Senior house officer
RCST	Regional Committee on Specialist Training	**SI**	International System of Units
RCT	Root canal treatment	**SLE**	Systemic lupus erythematosus
Retics	Reticulocytes		
RBBB	Right bundle branch block	**SMV**	Submentovertex (radiograph)
RF	Rheumatoid factor *or* rheumatoid fever	**SOA**	Swelling of ankles
		SOB	Shortness of breath
RFH	Right femoral hernia	**SOL**	Space-occupying lesion (usually neoplasm)
RFT	Renal function tests		
Rh	Rhesus	**SR**	Senior Registrar
RHA	Regional Health Authority	**SRN**	Staff Registered Nurse
		SS	Sjögren's syndrome *or* systemic sclerosis *or* sagittal split (osteotomy)
RhF	Rheumatic fever		
RHF	Right heart failure		
RIF	Right iliac fossa		
ROU	Recurrent oral ulcers	**ST**	Segment of ECG record
RPA	Radiation Protection Advisor	**STD**	Sexually transmitted diseases
RPCFT	Reiter protein complement fixation test	**SVC**	Superior vena cava
		SVD	Spontaneous vaginal delivery
RPS	Radiation Protection Supervisor	**Svh**	Sievherts
RRF	Retrograde root filling		
RTA	Road traffic accident	**T**	Temperature *or* wave on ECG
RVF	Right ventricular failure		
		TASS	Technical and supervisory staff section
SA	Subarachnoid		
SAC	Standing Advisory Committee (of JCHTD)	**TB**	Tuberculosis
		TFT	Thyroid function tests
		TI	Tricuspid incompetence
SBE	Subacute bacterial endocarditis	**TIBC**	Total iron binding capacity
SC	Subcutaneous	**TLC**	Tender loving care *or* total lung capacity
SCOPME	Standing Committee on Postgraduate Medical Education in England	**TLE**	Temporal lobe epilepsy
		TMJ	Temporomandibular joint
SERC	Science and Engineering Research Council	**TPHA**	Treponema pallidum haemagglutination (test)
SG	Specific gravity		
SGGT	*see* GGT	**TPI**	Treponema pallidum immobilisation (test)
SGOT	*see* AST		

TPN	Total parenteral nutrition	**USDAW**	Union of Shop, Distributive and Allied Workers
TPR	Temperature, pulse, respiration	**UTI**	Urinary tract infection
TRH	Thyroid-releasing hormone		
TS	Tricuspid stenosis	**VC**	Vital capacity
TSH	Thyroid-stimulating hormone	**VDRL**	Venereal Disease Research Laboratories (test)
TSSU	Theatre sterile supplies unit		
		VF	Ventricular fibrillation
		VSD	Ventricular septal defect
		VSS	Vertical subsigmoid
UC	Ulcerative colitis	**VV**	Varicose veins
U&E	Urea and electrolytes	**VZV**	Varicella zoster virus
UGS	Urogenital system		
UHA	University Hospitals Association	**WBC**	White blood count
UMN	Upper motor neurone	**WCC**	White cell count
URTI	Upper respiratory tract infection	**WR**	Wasserman reaction

Other terminology

$100\frac{120}{80}60$: Blood pressure: standing 120/80 (systolic/diastolic); lying 100/60

nocte: in the night
mane: in the morning
2°: Metastasis
#: Fracture
5 LICSMCL: Usually refers to apex beat situation: in the 5th left intercostal space in the mid-clavicular line
stat: immediately
bd: twice daily (*bis die*)
qds, qid: four times daily (*quater die sumendum, quater in die*)
tds: three times daily (*ter die sumendum*)
prn: as required (*pro re nata*)
BTS: Reflexes: biceps, triceps, supinator
KAP: Reflexes: knee, ankle, plantar
Babinski reflex = plantar reflex
Koch's infection = tuberculosis
Specific infection = syphilis
Mitotic lesion = malignant neoplasm
Lymphoproliferative state = sometimes used instead of 'leukaemia'
Special Clinic = clinic for sexually transmitted diseases
Vital signs = temperature, blood pressure, pulse, respiration
Inoculation risk = patient infected with HBV or HIV

♀	–	Female
♂	–	Male
1°	–	Primary
2°	–	Secondary
>	–	Great than
<	–	Lesser than
≥	–	Greater than or equal to
≤	–	Less than or equal to
+	–	Positive
−	–	Negative
↑	–	Increased
↓	–	Decreased

Appendix 2 Cephalometric points and planes

Anterior nasal spine (ANS): The tip of the anterior nasal spine

Articulare (Ar): The projection on a lateral skull radiograph of the posterior outline of the condylar process on to the interior outline of the cranial base

Glabella: The most prominent point over the frontal bone

Gnathion (Gn): The most anterior inferior point of the bony chin

Gonion (Go): The most posterior inferior point at the angle of the mandible

Menton (Me): The most inferior point on the bony chin

Nasion (N): The most anterior point on the frontonasal suture

Orbitale (Or): The lowest point on the bony margin of the orbit

Pogonion (Pog): The most anterior point on the bony chin

Point A: The deepest point on the maxillary profile between the anterior nasal spine and the alveolar crest

Point B: The deepest point on the mandibular profile between the pogonion and the alveolar crest

Porion (Po): The uppermost, outermost point on the bony external acoustic meatus

Posterior nasal spine (PNS): The tip of the posterior nasal spine

Sella (S): The mid-point of the sella turcica

Frankfort plane: The plane through the orbitale and porion. This is meant to approximate the horizontal plane when the head is in the free postural position but this varies appreciably (substitutes for maxillary plane on clinical examination)

Mandibular plane: The plane through the gonion and menton

Maxillary plane: The plane through ANS and PNS (substitutes for Frankfort plane on clinical examination).

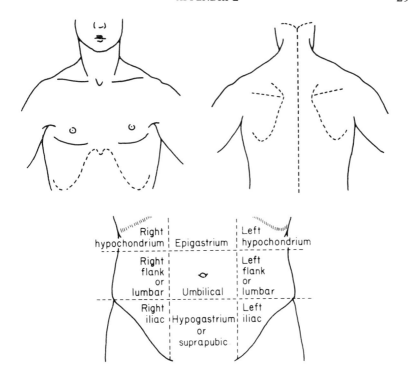

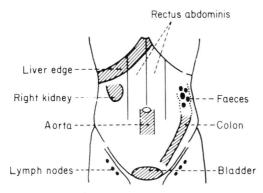

Palpation of the abdomen: some normal findings.

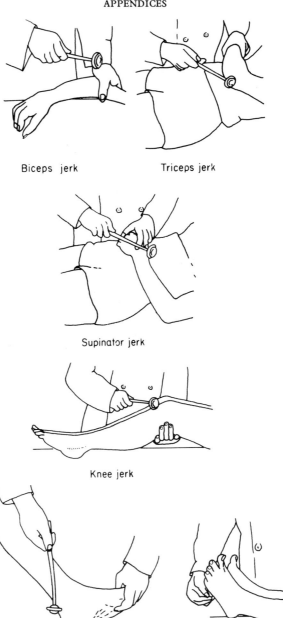

Biceps jerk

Triceps jerk

Supinator jerk

Knee jerk

Ankle jerk

Plantar reflex

Reflexes.

Appendix 3 Some qualifications in dentistry and medicine

BA	Bachelor of Arts
BCh	Bachelor of Surgery
BChD	Bachelor of Dental Surgery
BDS	Bachelor of Dental Surgery
BS	Bachelor of Surgery
BSc	Bachelor of Science
ChM	Master of Surgery
Dip Bact	Diploma in Bacteriology
DA	Diploma in Anaesthetics
DCH	Diploma in Child Health
DDPH	Diploma in Dental Public Health
DDR	Diploma in Dental Radiology
DDS	Diploma in Dental Science (*or* Doctor of Dental Science/Surgery
DLO	Diploma in Laryngology and Otology
DOrth	Diploma in Orthodontics
DMRD	Diploma in Medical Radiodiagnosis
DPhil	Doctor of Philosophy
DPM	Diploma in Psychological Medicine
DRCOG	Diploma of Royal College of Obstetricians and Gynaecologists
DRD	Diploma in Restorative Dentistry
DSc	Doctor of Science
DTM + H	Diploma in Tropical Medicine and Hygiene
FDS	Fellow in Dental Surgery (FDS, RCS, FDS RCPS, FDS RCSE)
FFARCS	Fellow in Faculty of Anaesthesia, Royal College of Surgeons
FFCM	Fellow in Faculty of Community Medicine
FFD	Fellow in Faculty of Dental Surgery
FFR	Fellow in Faculty of Radiology
FRCGP	Fellow of Royal College of General Practitioners
FRCOG	Fellow of Royal College of Obstetricians and Gynaecologists
FRCP	Fellow of Royal College of Physicians
FRCPath	Fellow of Royal College of Pathologists
FRCPsych	Fellow of Royal College of Psychiatrists
FRCS	Fellow of Royal College of Surgeons
LDS	Licentiate in Dental Surgery
LRCP	Licentiate of Royal College of Physicians
LRCS	Licentiate of Royal College of Surgeons
MA	Master of Arts
MB	Bachelor of Medicine
MCCD	Membership in Clinical Community Dentistry
MD	Doctor of Medicine
MDS	Master in Dental Surgery
MGDS	Membership in General Dental Surgery
MOrth	Master in Orthodontics
MPhil	Master of Philosophy
MRCGP	Member of Royal College of General Practitioners
MRCOG	Member of Royal College of Obstetricians and Gynaecologists
MRCP	Member of Royal College of Physicians

MRCPath	Member of the Royal College of Pathologists
MRCPsych	Member of the Royal College of Psychiatrists
MRCS	Member of the Royal College of Surgeons
MS	Master of Surgery (in USA, Master of Science)
MSc	Master of Science
PhD	Doctor of Philosophy

Appendix 4 US-accepted abbreviations

aa	Of each	B-K	Below knee (amputation)
abd	Abdomen	bm	Bowel movement
ABGs	Arterial blood gases	B/M	Black male
ac	Before meals	bp	Blood pressure
ACC	Ambulatory Care Center	BPH	Benign prostatic hypertrophy
ADL	Activities of daily living	BRP	Bathroom privileges
ad lib	Freely	BS	Blood sugars
AF	Atrial fibrillation	BSO	Bilateral salpingo-oophorectomy
AFB	Acid fast bacillus		
AFO	Ankle foot orthosis	BSP	Bromsulfalein test
A/G	Albumin/globulin ratio	BUN	Blood urea nitrogen
AI	Aortic insufficiency	Bx	Biopsy
A-K	Above knee (amputation)		
alb	Albumin		
ALL	Acute lymphocytic leukemia	c	With
am	In the morning	CA	Carcinoma
AMA	Against medical advice	CABG	Coronary artery bypass graft
amb	Ambulation		
AMI	Acute myocardial infarction	CAD	Coronary artery disease
		Cal	Calorie
Angio	Angiology	cap	capsule
AODM	Adult onset diabetes mellitus	CAPD	Continued ambulatory peritoneal dialysis
A & P	Anterior and posterior (repair)	CBC	Complete blood count, excluding red cell count
AP	Apical pulse		
AROM	Active range of motion	cc	Chief complaint
AS	Aortic stenosis	cc	cubic centimeter
ASHD	Arteriosclerotic heart disease	CCU	Coronary Care Unit
		CHF	Congestive heart failure
As Tol	As tolerated	cho	Carbohydrate
ATC	Around the clock	CLL	Chronic lymphatic leukemia
A&W	Alive and well		
		CNS	Central nervous system
		c/o	Complaining of
		COPD	Chronic obstructive pulmonary disease
BE	Barium enema		
Bee	Basal energy expenditure	CPM	Continued passive motion
B/F	Black female	cr	Creatinine
bid	Twice a day	CRF	Chronic renal failure
biw	Twice a week	CSF	Cerebral spinal fluid

CT	Computerized tomography	**FBS**	Fasting blood sugar
CVA	Cerebrovascular accident	**FUO**	Fever of unknown origin
CVP	Central venous pressure	**Fx**	Fracture
Cx	Cervix		
Cysto	Cystoscopy	**GB**	Gallbladder
		Gc	Gonorrhea
		GI	Gastrointestinal
DASU	Day Ambulatory Surgery Unit	**gm**	Gram
		gr	Grain
D/c	Discontinue	**grav**	gravida
D & C	Dilatation and curettage	**gtt**	Drop
		GU	Genito-urinary
DDD	Pacemaker (type of)	**Gyn**	Gynecology
Diff	WBC differential	**GTT**	Glucose tolerance test
Dig	Digitalis		
DM	Diabetes mellitus		
D/O	Diet order	**HA**	Headache
DOA	Dead on arrival	**HAA**	Hyperalimentation
DOE	Dyspnea on exertion	**Hb**	Hemoglobin
DSA	Digital subtraction angiography	**HBP**	High blood pressure
		HCTZ	Hydrochlorothiazide
D/T	Due to	**HCVD**	Hypertensive cardiovascular disease
DTR	Deep tendon reflex		
DTs	Delirium tremens	**HEENT**	Head, ears, eyes, nose and throat
DUB	Dysfunctional uterine bleeding		
		hgt	Height
DVT	Deep vein thrombosis	**HHB**	Hand held nebulizer
Dx	Diagnosis	**H & N**	Head and neck
		HO	House Officer
		HOH	Hard of hearing
ECG	Electrocardiogram	**H & P**	History and physical
EEG	Electroencephalogram	**HP**	Hot packs
EENT	Eyes, ears, nose and throat	**hr**	Hour
		hs	At bedtime
EKG	Electrocardiogram	**HTN**	Hypertension
EMG	Electromyogram	**Hx**	History
ENT	Ears, nose and throat		
EOM	Extraocular movements		
ER	Emergency Room	**IBW**	Ideal body weight
ERCP	Endoscopic retrograde cholangiopancreato-graphy	**ICP**	Intracranial pressure
		ICU	Intensive Care Unit
		I & D	Incision and drainage
ESRD	End stage renal disease	**IF**	Injury factor
ETOH	Ethyl alcohol	**IM**	Intramuscularly
ETP	Elective termination of pregnancy	**I & O**	Intake and output
		IPD	Intermittent peritoneal dialysis
ex	Exercise		

IPPB	Intermittent positive pressure breathing	**m**	murmur
IUD	Intrauterine device	**MAE**	Moving all extremities
IUP	Intrauterine pregnancy	**max**	Maximal
IV	Intravenously	**mcg**	microgram
IVP	Intravenous pyelogram	**mEq**	Milliequivalent
		mgm	milligram
		MI	Myocardial infarct or if referring to valvular lesion, Mitral insufficiency
JODM	Juvenile onset diabetes mellitus	**MIC**	Medical Intensive Care
jt	Joint	**MICU**	Medical Intensive Care Unit
		min	Minimal
K	Potassium	**MMT**	Manual muscle test
Kg	Kilogram	**mod**	Moderate
KUB	Flat film of kidney, ureters, bladder	**MOM**	Milk of magnesia
		MOV	Multiple oral vitamin
		MR	Magnetic resonance
		MS	multiple sclerosis
L or l	Liter		
lab	Laboratory	**N/B**	Newborn
LBBB	Left bundle branch block	**NB**	Note well
		neg	negative
LBP	Low back pain	**NG**	Nasogastric
LE	Lower extremity	**nl**	normal
LFT	Liver function test	**NPO**	Nothing by mouth
LLB	Long leg brace	**N/S**	Normal saline
LLC	Long leg cast	**NSR**	Normal sinus rhythm
LLL	Left lower lobe	**Ntg**	Nitroglycerin
LLQ	Left lower quadrant	**N & V**	Nausea and vomiting
LMP	Last menstrual period		
LOA	Left occiput anterior		
LOP	Left occiput posterior	**OB**	Obstetrics
LOT	Left occiput transverse	**OD**	Right eye
LP	Lumbar puncture	**OHS**	Open heart surgery
LPN	Licensed Practical Nurse	**OOB**	Out of bed
		OPD	Outpatient Department
LS	Lumbosacral	**OR**	Operating room
LSSP	Lumbosacral spine and pelvis	**OS**	Left eye
		OT	Occupational therapy
Lt	Left	**OU**	Both eyes
LUL	Left upper lobe		
LUQ	Left upper quadrant		
LVF	Left ventricular failure	**P & A**	Percussion and auscultation
LVH	Left ventricular hypertrophy	**PAT**	Paroxysmal auricular tachycardia
Lytes	Electrolytes		

pc	after meals	**RLL**	Right lower lobe
PCA	Patient controlled	**RLQ**	Right lower quadrant
	analgesia	**RML**	Right middle lobe
PCM	Protein caloric	**R/O**	Rule out
	malnutrition	**ROA**	Right occiput anterior
PE	Physical examination	**ROM**	Range of motion
PEEP	Positive and expiration	**ROP**	Right occiput posterior
	pressure	**ROS**	Review of systems
PERRLA	Pupils equal, round,	**ROT**	Right occiput
	reactive to light and		transverse
	accommodation	**RROM**	Resisted range of
PH	Past history		motion
phys ther	Physical therapy	**rt**	Right
PLD	Pelvic inflammatory	**RT**	Radiation therapy
	disease	**RTC**	Return to Clinic
pm	In the evening	**Ru**	Retrograde urogram
PMD	Private physician	**RUL**	Right upper lobe
PMI	Point of maximal	**RUQ**	Right upper quadrant
	impulse		
PND	Post nasal drip		
PO	Postoperative	**s**	Without
Pos or +	Positive	S_1	First heart sound
PP	Post partum	S_2	Second heart sound
PPD	Purified protein	S_3	Third heart sound
	derivative	S_4	Fourth heart sound
PRBLs	Packed red blood cells	**SBE**	Subacute bacterial
PROM	Passive range of motion		endocarditis
prn	As necessary	**SBFT**	Small bowel follow
pro	Protein		through
PSP	Phenosulfonphthalein	**Sed rate**	Erythrocyte
PSVT	Paroxysmal		sedimentation rate
	supraventricular	**SICU**	Surgical Intensive Care
	tachycardia		Unit
PT	Physical Therapy	**Sig**	Directions
PT	Physiotherapy	**SLB**	Short leg brace
PTA	Prior to admission	**SLC**	Short leg cast
PVC	Premature ventricular	**SLE**	Systemic lupus
	contractions		erythematosus
PVD	Peripheral vascular	**SLR**	Straight leg raising
	disease	**S/M**	Statement
		SNF	Skilled Nursing Facility
		SOB	Shortness of breath
qd	Every day	**S/T**	States that
qid	Four times a day	**STD**	Sexually transmitted
qod	Every other day		disease
q2d	Every second day	**SUBQ**	Subcutaneous
RCU	Respiratory Care Unit		
RHD	Rheumatic heart	**TAH**	Total abdominal
	disease		hysterectomy

THR	Total hip replacement	**VA**	Visual acuity
tid	Three times a day	**VAcC**	Visual acuity with
TKR	Total knee replacement		correction
TM	Tympanic membrane	**VCsC**	Visual acuity without
TMJ	Temporal mandibular		correction
	joint	**VF**	Ventricular fibrillation
TPR	Temperature, pulse and	**vit/min**	vitamin/mineral
	respiration	**VNA**	Visiting Nurses'
TUR	Transurethral resection		Association
TKVO	To keep vein open	**vs**	vital signs
		VT	Ventricular tachycardia
U	Regarding		
U/A	Urinalysis	**WBC**	White blood count
UE	Upper extremity	**w/c**	Wheelchair
UGI	Upper gastrointestinal	**W/D**	Well-developed
U&L	Upper and lower	**W/F**	White female
URI	Upper respiratory	**WFL**	Within functional limits
	infection	**W/M**	White male
Urol	Urology	**W/N**	Well-nourished
US	Ultrasound	**WNL**	Within normal limits
USB	Ultrasonic nebulizer	**wt**	Weight
UTI	Urinary tract infection	**W/u**	Work-up

Appendix 5 Sterilisation in the dental surgery

Method	Temperature	Time	Comments
Autoclave	121°C at 15 lb/in² *or* 134°C at 32 lb/in²	15 minutes 3 minutes	Most efficient form of sterilisation for metal instruments and fabrics
Hot air oven	160°C *or* 180°C	60 minutes 20 minutes	Effective but time consuming and chars fabrics
Glutaraldehyde	20°C	60 minutes	Does *not* sterilise but kills most bacteria, spores and viruses. Useful for heat-sensitive equipment. Deteriorates rapidly with time

Appendix 6 Further reading

Calman KC. *Basic skills for surgical housemen*. Edinburgh: Churchill Livingstone, 1971.

Cawson RA, Spector RG. *Clinical pharmacology in dentistry*. Edinburgh: Churchill Livingstone, 1985.

Dental practitioners' formulary. London: British Dental Association.

Houston WJB, Isaacson KG. *Orthodontic treatment with removable appliances*. Bristol: Wrights, 1980.

Mason RA. *A guide to dental radiography* (Dental Practitioner Handbook No. 27). Bristol: Wrights, 1988.

Robinson RO. *Medical emergencies: diagnosis and management*. London: Heinemann, 1982.

Scully C, Cawson RA. *Medical problems in dentistry*. Bristol: Wrights, 1987.

Seear J. *Law and ethics in dentistry* (Dental Practitioner Handbook No. 19). Bristol: Wrights, 1975.

Zook EG. *The primary care of facial injuries*. Littleton, Massachusetts: PSG Publishing, 1980.

Index